Osteoporosis - Recent Advances, New Perspectives and Applications

Edited by Luis Rodrigo

Published in London, United Kingdom

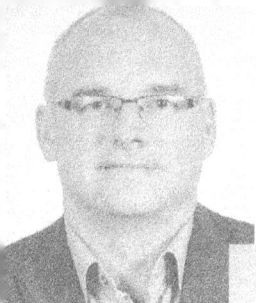
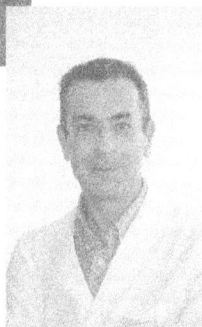
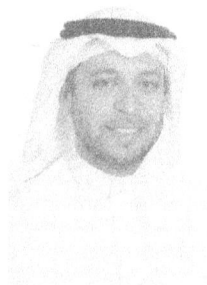
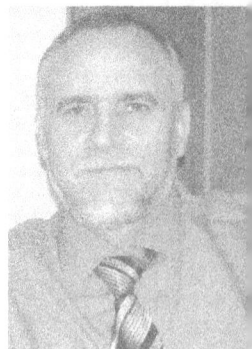
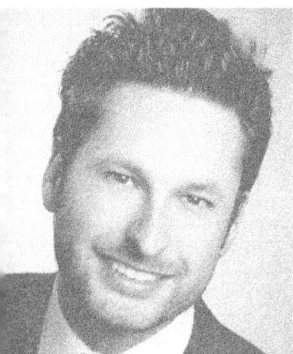
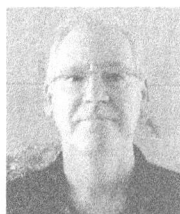
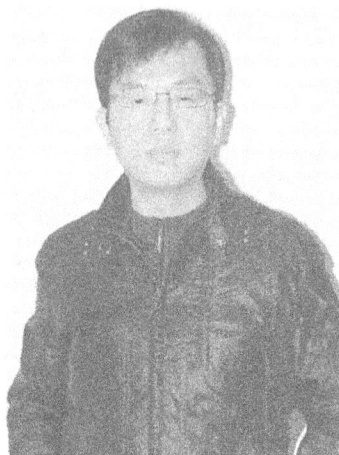

IntechOpen

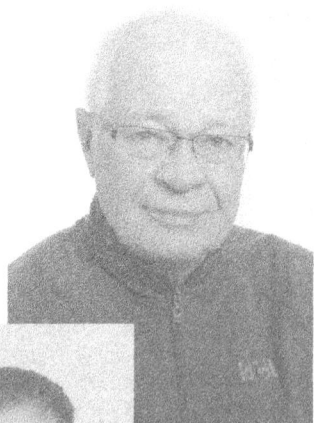
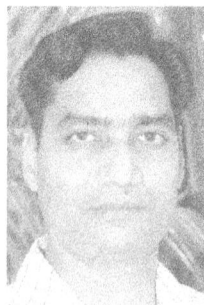
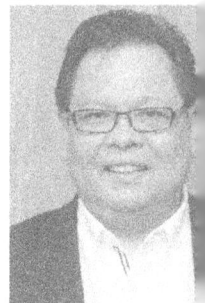
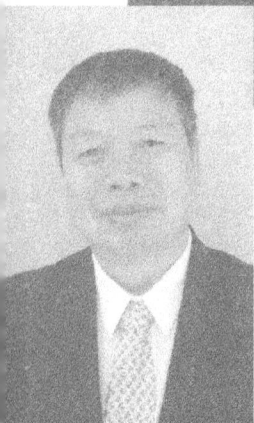
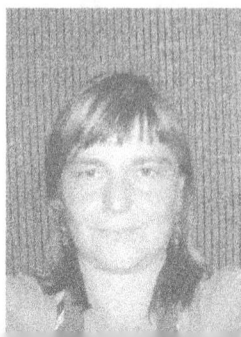
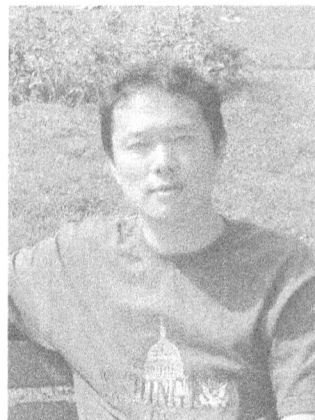

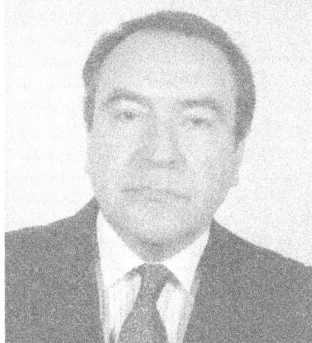

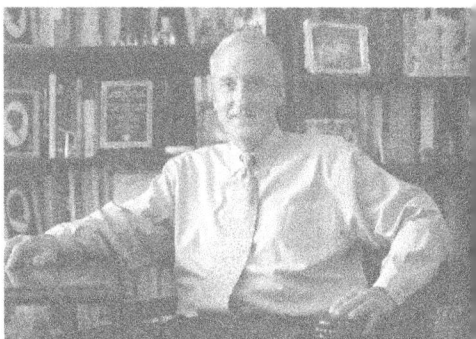

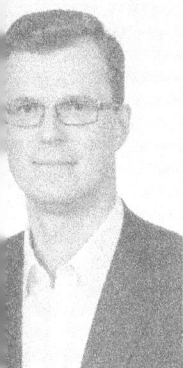

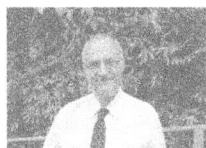

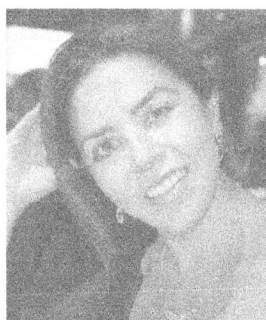

Supporting open minds since 2005

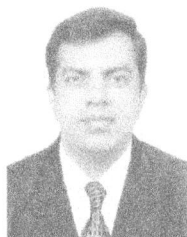

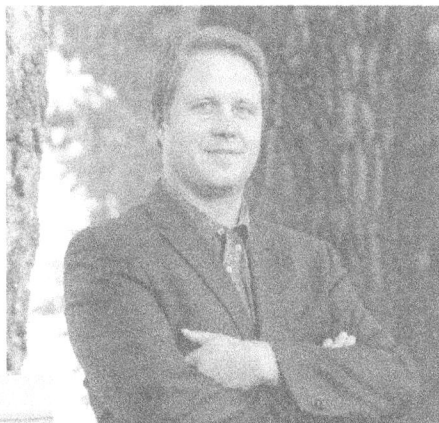

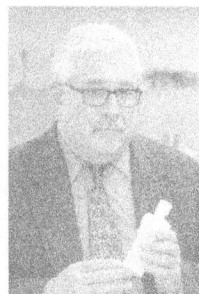

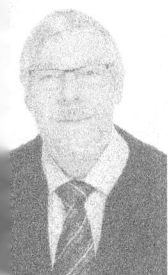

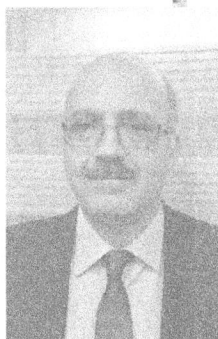

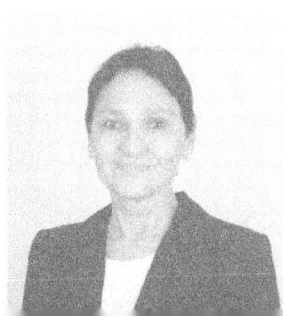

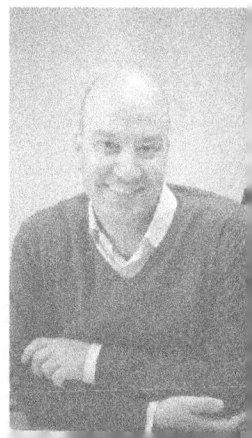

Osteoporosis - Recent Advances, New Perspectives and Applications
http://dx.doi.org/10.5772/intechopen.91509
Edited by Luis Rodrigo

Contributors
Sergio Luchini Batista, José Renan Vieira Da Costa Júnior, Olga Cvijanović Peloza, Sandra Pavičić Žeželj, Ivana Pavičić, Ana Terezija Jerbić Radetić, Sanja Zoričić Cvek, Jasna Lulić Drenjak, Gordana Starčević Klasan, Ariana Fužinac Smojver, Juraj Arbanas, Gordana Kenđel Jovanović, Rajeev Aurora, Di Wu, Anna Cline-Smith, Elena Shashkova, Plauto C. A. Watanabe, Giovani Antonio Rodrigues, Fabio Santos Bottacin, Rafael Angelo Soares Vieira, Enéas de Almeida Souza Filho, Michel Campos Ribeiro, Rodrigues Azenha Rodrigues Azenha, Luis Rodrigo

Notice
Statements and opinions expressed in the chapters are these of the individual contributors and not necessarily those of the editors or publisher. No responsibility is accepted for the accuracy of information contained in the published chapters. The publisher assumes no responsibility for any damage or injury to persons or property arising out of the use of any materials, instructions, methods or ideas contained in the book.

First published in London, United Kingdom, 2021 by IntechOpen
IntechOpen is the global imprint of INTECHOPEN LIMITED, registered in England and Wales, registration number: 11086078, 5 Princes Gate Court, London, SW7 2QJ, United Kingdom
Printed in Croatia

British Library Cataloguing-in-Publication Data
A catalogue record for this book is available from the British Library

Additional hard and PDF copies can be obtained from orders@intechopen.com

Osteoporosis - Recent Advances, New Perspectives and Applications
Edited by Luis Rodrigo
p. cm.
Print ISBN 978-1-83969-236-9
Online ISBN 978-1-83969-237-6
eBook (PDF) ISBN 978-1-83969-238-3

We are IntechOpen,
the world's leading publisher of
Open Access books
Built by scientists, for scientists

5,300+
Open access books available

131,000+
International authors and editors

155M+
Downloads

Our authors are among the

156
Countries delivered to

Top 1%
most cited scientists

12.2%
Contributors from top 500 universities

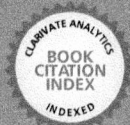

Interested in publishing with us?
Contact book.department@intechopen.com

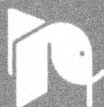

Meet the editor

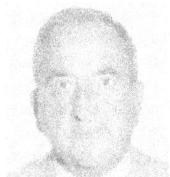

Dr. Luis Rodrigo, MD, was a Professor of Medicine at the University of Oviedo, Spain. He obtained a Ph.D. in 1975 and has developed a long teaching and research career over 42 years. To date, he has published 704 scientific papers, 422 of which are written in English and the rest in Spanish. He has been the main investigator in 45 clinical trials and has directed 40 doctoral theses. He has published 42 chapters in books on several subjects and has edited 32 books in his specialty. His areas of interest are celiac disease and Autoimmune diseases, *Helicobacter pylori*, chronic HCV infections, and other types of infectious diseases.

Contents

Preface   XI

Chapter 1   1
Introductory Chapter: Osteoporosis Overview
by Luis Rodrigo

Chapter 2   13
Glucocorticoid-Induced Osteoporosis
by José Renan Vieira da Costa Júnior and Sérgio Luchini Batista

Chapter 3   29
Osteoporosis and Dietary Inflammatory Index
by Olga Cvijanović Peloza, Sandra Pavičić Žeželj, Gordana Kenđel Jovanović,
Ivana Pavičić, Ana Terezija Jerbić Radetić, Sanja Zoričić Cvek,
Jasna Lulić Drenjak, Gordana Starčević Klasan, Ariana Fužinac Smojver
and Juraj Arbanas

Chapter 4   43
Osteoporosis: A Multifactorial Disease
by Di Wu, Anna Cline-Smith, Elena Shashkova and Rajeev Aurora

Chapter 5   61
Bone Quality of the Dento-Maxillofacial Complex and Osteoporosis.
Opportunistic Radiographic Interpretation
by Plauto Christopher Aranha Watanabe, Giovani Antonio Rodrigues,
Marcelo Rodrigues Azenha, Michel Campos Ribeiro,
Enéas de Almeida Souza Filho, Rafael Angelo Soares Vieira
and Fabio Santos Bottacin

Preface

Osteoporosis is a significant social health problem, not only in terms of pain and disability but also in terms of mortality rate. Osteoporosis affects approximately 200 million people worldwide, with nearly 9 million fractures occurring annually.

This disease is defined by a generalized and progressive reduction in both bone mineral and bone matrix, which results in a bone of normal composition but decreased mass. Functionally, osteoporotic bone is characterized by greater fragility and an increased propensity to fracture. Osteoporosis ranks as the most common metabolic bone disease and the most common skeletal disorder in the world. As such, it constitutes a major public health problem. Despite heightened awareness among patients and clinicians alike, and the availability of efficacious anti-osteoporosis medications, osteoporosis is still underdiagnosed and undertreated.

Metabolic syndrome, together with major obesity and diabetes mellitus, is associated with osteoporosis, and all of these conditions have become major global health problems over the last decades. The interaction between obesity and bone metabolism is complex and not fully understood. Several mechanical, biochemical, and hormonal mechanisms have been proposed to explain the association between adipose tissue and bone. Low-grade systemic inflammation is probably harmful to the bone and increased bone marrow adipogenesis may lead to decreased bone mass in obese individuals.

A better understanding of the association between adipose and bone tissue may help to identify new molecular therapeutic targets that will promote osteoblastic activity and/or inhibit adipogenesis and osteoclastic activity. An analysis of the medical literature shows clearly that male osteoporosis is underscreened, underdiagnosed, and undertreated, both in primary and secondary prevention of fragility fractures.

In the introductory chapter, Dr. Rodrigo provides an update on the state of the art of osteoporosis in clinical practice.

The next chapter describes glucocorticoid-induced osteoporosis. It examines its main characteristics, frequency, and treatment and prevention options.

The next chapter examines the relationship between osteoporosis and diet. The authors comment on the role of inflammatory factors in food and they recommend the consumption of an anti-inflammatory diet to treat and prevent osteoporosis.

In the next chapter, the authors describe the diverse factors that can contribute to osteoporosis with an emphasis on the disease's multifactorial nature and therapeutic consequences.

The routine study of the dental maxillofacial complex including the performance of panoramic radiological pictures is a good method for detection of osteoporosis in early-stage and helps to stop its progression for the rest of bone structures of the body. This is described in the last chapter.

One interesting and sometimes forgotten aspect is the effect of osteoporosis on the dento-maxillofacial complex. In this case, panoramic radiographies can be used for the evaluation of healthy dental structure and maintenance.

Osteoporosis is called the 'silent disease' because although it does not give significant symptoms when it is not complicated, it can cause fragility fractures with serious consequences and even death. Furthermore, the consequences of osteoporosis have been calculated to weigh heavily on the costs of health systems in all countries. Osteoporosis is considered a female disease. The hormonal changes that occur after menopause certainly contribute to a significant risk of osteoporosis and fractures in women. However, while there is no doubt that women are more exposed to osteoporosis and fragility fractures, the literature clearly indicates that physicians tend to underestimate osteoporosis in men.

Bisphosphonates are standard medicine for the treatment of osteoporosis and have been innovated to overcome complicated rules for their appropriate administration or poor intestinal absorption. Weekly, as well as monthly oral bisphosphonates, are available. Furthermore, we are now allowed to choose intravenous administration of bisphosphonates for osteoporosis. Good persistence and adherence are critical and essential issues to address to achieve the aim of osteoporosis treatment with bisphosphonates. Variable formulations of bisphosphonate are now able to bring patients closer to reduced rates of fragile fracture due to osteoporosis.

Detection of osteoporosis, as a multifactorial disease, and its clinical consequence of bone fracture, has been the subject of extensive research. Recent advances in machine learning have enabled the field of artificial intelligence to make impressive breakthroughs in complex data environments where the human capacity to identify high-dimensional relationships is limited. The field of osteoporosis is one such domain, notwithstanding technical and clinical concerns regarding the application of electronic methods.

Luis Rodrigo MD
Professor of Medicine,
University of Oviedo,
Oviedo, Asturias, Spain

Chapter 1

Introductory Chapter: Osteoporosis Overview

Luis Rodrigo

1. Introduction

Osteoporosis is a skeletal disease, characterized by a thinning of the bone (loss of bone mass), accompanied by a deterioration of its internal architecture that compromises its resistance, producing a greater fragility of the bones and an increased risk of fractures. The most affected bones are especially those of the spine and hip, although any bone in the body can be involved. As the main risk factor for suffering bone fragility fractures, which increases with age, it is an important public health problem that has undoubted social, health and economic repercussions; but above all it causes pain, functional limitation and severe alteration in people's quality of life.

The World Health Organization (WHO) defines it mainly in women as "the presence of a bone mineral density (BMD) less than or equal to 2.5 standard deviations below the average bone mass of healthy 20-year-olds", which is carried performed using a specific radiological test, called bone mineral densitometry. Since bone loss often occurs without symptoms, osteoporosis is often considered a "silent disease" that can occur in both sexes and increases with age. As bone tissue deteriorates, together with the architecture changes, the bone becomes so weak, that a relatively minor bump or fall, causes a vertebra to fracture or break. That is, the clinical manifestations of osteoporosis appear as a consequence of its complications, which are spontaneous fractures or after minimal trauma. Many environmental factors are involved in their onset [1].

However, there is a risk of considering that the loss of bone mass, causes only musculoskeletal pain. Women are more susceptible to suffering from bone fractures, as direct consequences of this disease, due to the fact that faced with a calcium deficiency in the diet, together with a vitamin D deficiency, during pregnancy and lactation, the body goes to diminish the reserves of calcium in the bone, which is the cause of gradual loss of bone mass. For this reason, its appearance is later and more frequently in amenorrheic or post-menopausal women, who also have a decrease in the production of estrogens by the ovaries and other hormonal deficiencies that affect metabolism in the bone. Factors that increase the risk of developing osteoporosis are calcium and vitamin D deficiencies due to malnutrition, sedentary life or lack of physical activity, and tobacco and/or alcohol consumption. Other secondary causes have been reported, such as celiac disease, monoclonal gammopathy of uncertain origin, chronic renal failure, diabetes mellitus, and renal tubular acidosis. Some epigenetic factors can be associated [2].

The best strategy for treating osteoporosis, is the prevention. Bone, or bone tissue, is a very dynamic living tissue throughout life, which is constantly formed (ossification), grows and remodels (bone turnover). For these processes (formation, growth and remodeling), important for the integrity or strength of the bone, hormonal activities, certain nutrients (calcium, phosphorus, magnesium, vitamin D, vitamin K) and physical activity take part. Therefore, they are recognized as factors that play an important role in the prevention and treatment of osteoporosis. You have to get a good BMD and maintain it throughout your life. For this, it is necessary to achieve optimal bone formation in the youngest and then avoid loss of bone mass in adulthood and old age.

To achieve these goals, it is necessary to carry out a diet that provides the essential nutrients for the formation, growth and maintenance of bones. It is important to guarantee the consumption of the daily needs or minimum requirements of Calcium (1300 mg/day), Phosphorus (1250 mg/day), Magnesium (420 mg/day) and Vitamin D (20 mcg/day equivalent to 800 IU/day), through normal nutrition (daily consumption of foods that contain these nutrients) or supplementation. Perform appropriate physical exercise for each age through frequent outdoor activity, which ensures prudent sun exposure, for the synthesis of vitamin D in the skin, but avoiding overexposure, due to the risks it has on skin health [3–5].

2. Classification

Taking into account the causes that produce it, osteoporosis can be classified as primary and secondary.

2.1 Primary or involutive

It is the most common type of osteoporosis. This diagnosis is established after evaluating the patient, when the cause/s that can be related, are not found. In turn, primary osteoporosis can in turn be subdivided into juvenile, postmenopausal, age-related, and idiopathic forms.

2.2 Secondary osteoporosis

When the loss of bone mass is caused by another disease, or by the use of particular drugs. Fractures occur most frequently at the level of the hip bones, vertebrae of the spine, and wrist. Vertebral fractures can cause loss of height of the spine as a whole and deformity of the rib cage.

Depending on the results obtained in BMD, the results can be classified according to the T scale, which refers to the mean bone density of the healthy population of the same sex and 20 years of age in the following categories:

2.3 Normal

When bone mineral density is greater than −1 standard deviation (SD) on the T scale.

2.4 Osteopenia

When the BMD presents a standard deviation between 0 to −1, on the T scale. This variety is not included in osteoporosis and generally does not require drug treatment.

2.5 Osteoporosis

If bone mineral density is less than −2.5 standard deviations on the T scale.

2.6 Established osteoporosis

When there is osteoporosis and it has caused a fracture [6, 7].

3. Epidemiology

Osteoporosis and its related complications, are one of the main health problems in the world. This disease is estimated to affect at least to 200 million of women globally and is a major cause of morbidity and mortality. Among North American postmenopausal white women, 57% are osteopenic and 30% osteoporotic, and from the age of 80 ahead, 27% of women present osteopenia and 70% osteoporosis, with a large increase in the latter.

It is reported that approximately 40% of white US women and 13% of white US men in their 50s will experience at least one brittle bone fracture in their lifetime. It is also estimated that 1 in 3 women and 1 in 12 men over the age of 50 suffer from osteoporosis. And it is responsible for millions of fractures annually, many of which include the lumbar vertebrae [8, 9].

4. Etiology

The bones of the body are subjected to continuous remodeling through processes of formation and reabsorption, they also serve as the body's calcium reservoir. From the age of 35, the loss of bone mass begins. Multiple diseases or sedentary lifestyles, can increase the bone loss causing osteoporosis at an earlier age.

The main mechanisms that cause osteoporosis are: 1/. Lack of sufficient bone mass, during the growth process. 2/. Excessive bone resorption mediated by osteoclasts. 3/. Inadequated new bone formation by osteoblasts, during the continuous process of bone renewal.

Menopause is the main cause of osteoporosis in women, due to the decrease in the production of estrogen hormones, which are reduced by physiological menopause or by surgical removal of the ovaries, causing rapid bone loss. Women, especially Caucasian and Asian, have lower bone mass than men. Bone loss results in decreased bone strength, easily leading to wrist, spine, and hip fractures.

However, there are a considerable number of causes of osteoporosis at any age that are not usually recognized or valued, but that can be identified if the patient undergoes an appropriated evaluation. Among them, the most common are undiagnosed Celiac Disease, due to the fact that it occurs frequently in a subclinical or asymptomatic way, and in people with negative antibody tests, untreated Non-Celiac Gluten Sensitivity, Monoclonal Gammapathy of uncertain significance, patients with Chronic Renal Failure, Diabetes Mellitus, and with Renal Tubular Acidosis.

In people with Celiac Disease or Non-Celiac Gluten Sensitivity without diagnosing, or following a gluten-free diet, the causes of both osteoporosis and osteopenia, are not limited to the existence of possible nutritional deficiencies, but may be due to processes inflammatory or autoimmune diseases in which the consumption of gluten can cause the development of autoantibodies.

The causes of secondary osteoporosis can be divided into several groups: endocrinological, gastrointestinal, by drugs, the presence of prolonged amenorrhea, or by various malignant tumor processes.

4.1 Endocrinological

Hyperthyroidism Hyperparathyroidism, Cushing's Syndrome, Type 1 Diabetes (insulin-dependent), Addison's disease, Sarcoidosis, Hypogonadism, Gigantism.

4.2 Gastrointestinal

Celiac disease, Ulcerative Colitis, Crohn's disease, Liver disease (especially Primary Biliary Cholangitis), Gastrectomy and Intestinal resection.

4.3 Drugs

The most frequently implicated are corticosteroids, lithium salts and some anti-epileptics, among others.

4.4 Various processes

Prolonged malnutrition, Large intestinal resections, Chronic alcoholism, Rheumatoid arthritis, Prolonged immobilization, others [10].

5. Clinical symptoms

Osteoporosis usually does not cause any symptoms. For this reason, it has been called the "silent epidemic". However, the error of considering that the loss of bone mass causes musculoskeletal pain is widespread. and patients are frequently referred to a specialist for this reason with suspected osteoporosis, especially pre-menopausal women or in young people.

The main clinical manifestations of osteoporosis are due to its complications, such as fractures, which mainly occur in the spine, wrists and hips. They are caused by minor trauma, such as a simple fall. This is why they are called "brittle fractures." They are usually classified broadly as "vertebral" and "non-vertebral." They produce the same symptoms as other fractures in the same location and are characterized by the presence of pain, deformity and functional impotence.

Vertebral fractures are the most frequent. They appear as a result of an effort, when carrying weights or bending over, but they can also appear spontaneously, without finding an apparent reason. They are typically accompanied by acute pain, which increases with movement and decreases with rest. The intensity of the pain usually decreases after the first 2–3 weeks and disappears in some cases after more than two years.

However, about two-thirds of vertebral fractures do not cause symptoms and can only be verified by radiography of the thoracic or lumbar spine. In some patients, as a consequence of structural alterations of the spine, instability of the spine may develop which is accompanied by muscle contractures and ligament tension, which can cause chronic pain.

The most serious fractures are those of the hip, usually as a result of a fall. Although there is no data to confirm this, the popular belief has spread that as a result of significant osteoporosis, the patient fractures the hip while standing and then falls, although this is not always the case [11].

6. Diagnosis

Osteoporosis is diagnosed by the evaluation of the findings of bone mineral densitometry test, which measures the amount of bone mass in the skeleton.

Its measurement is usually carried out at the level of the central skeleton (lumbar spine and/or neck of the femur) using specific radiology equipment (dual-DXA radiological densitometry). In the event that the central skeleton cannot be measured due to the existence of advanced osteoarthritis, fractures or prostheses that would invalidate the result, densitometry can be performed in such cases on the forearm or heel with other equipment (peripheral measurement DXA or quantitative ultrasonometry).

To evaluate the possible secondary causes of osteoporosis, basic and complementary tests are carried out; the latter, depending on the clinical suspicion:

7. Basic tests

1/. Comprehensive, complete and detailed medical history. 2/. Complete blood count with count of the three series, leukocyte formula and sedimentation rate. 3/. Coagulation study, to see if it is normal, or is accompanied by some alterations. 4/. Complete Biochemistry study, including serum levels of calcium, phosphorus, creatinine, alkaline phosphatase, sodium, and potassium. 5/. Serum levels of TSH and vitamin D. 6/. Total protein and albumin levels, with associated proteinogram to detect possible presence of gammapathies [12].

8. Supplementary tests

a. Determination of serum levels of parathormone, bone-specific alkaline phosphatase, prolactin and immunoglobulins.

b. Quantification of IgA, IgG and IgM immunoglobulins.

c. Determination of celiac disease antibodies (anti-transglutaminase IgA)

d. Biochemical markers of bone remodeling, such as the C-terminal propeptide of type I procollagen.

e. Fasting serum T3, T4 and plasma cortisol levels.

f. 24-hour urine study, to quantify total calcium and phosphorus elimination in one total day

g. Gastroscopy with taking duodenal biopsies to study celiac disease

h. Determination of insulin growth factor type 1 (in cases of anorexia and diabetes)

i. Fibroblast growth factor 23 levels

j. Bone biopsies samples, only when considered necessary in special cases

9. Treatments

The first step before recommending a treatment is to evaluate the patient for determining if its case belongs to primary or secondary osteoporosis, in order to detect the diseases that cause it, some of which often go unnoticed. If the causative disease is adequately treated and low bone density for age persists, treatment will depend on the dynamics of the bones.

The general guidelines are based on recommending an adequate amount of calcium in the diet, the practice of physical exercise and the use of medications that contribute to the maintenance or increase of bone mass. The main drugs used are calcium salts alone or associated with vitamin D, bisphosphonates, strontium ranelate, raloxifene and teriparatide, denosumab, calcitonin and hormonal treatment with estrogens.

Bisphosphonates are the most widely used group of drugs. Within these drugs are alendronic acid (alendronate), risedronate and ibandronate.

10. Diet, calcium and vitamin D supplements

Calcium is necessary to support bone growth, bone repair, and for maintaining the bone strength and is one of the main pillars of osteoporosis treatment. Calcium intake recommendations vary depending on the country and age. For individuals at high risk of osteoporosis over the age of 50, the amount recommended by the US Health Agencies is 1,200 mg per day. Calcium supplements can be used to increase dietary intake, and their absorption is optimized by taking several small (500 mg or less) dosages throughout the day.

The role of calcium in preventing and treating osteoporosis is unclear because some populations with extremely low intakes of calcium have low rates of bone fracture, and others with a high intake of calcium through both milk and its derivatives have a lot of bone fracture.

Other factors, such as protein intake, salt, vitamin D, exercise, sun exposure, also influence bone mineralization, making calcium intake one of many factors in the development of osteoporosis. Some studies show that a large intake of vitamin D, reduces the risk of fractures. However, other researchers have not confirmed these conclusions, so this aspect of treatment is a matter of debate [13].

Vegan diets can cause significant nutritional deficiencies, including calcium and vitamin D. These people tend to have low bone mass. The European Prospective Study on Cancer and Nutrition (EPIC, published in 2007) concludes that vegans have a 30% higher risk of bone fractures, than meat, fish and other subtypes of vegetarians, probably due to their considerably lower average consumption of calcium, although those who consume adequate amounts of this mineral have the same risk of fracture as the general population.

The risks of nutritional deficiencies and serious health consequences are especially important during pregnancy, in babies and in children. These deficiencies can only be prevented by choosing fortified foods or taking regular dietary supplements, for which personalized education and evaluation by nutrition professionals is essential. Both parents and adolescents may lack the necessary knowledge for proper vegan diet planning.

11. Physical exercise

Multiple studies confirm that maintaining an ideal weight and periodical performing aerobic physical exercise or resistance exercises, can maintain or increase bone density (DO) in postmenopausal women. Many researchers have evaluated which types of exercise are the most effective in improving BD and other measures of bone quality, however results vary [14].

One year of regular exercise increases bone density and proximal tibial moment of inertia in normal postmenopausal women. Walking, gymnastic training, stepping, jumping, endurance, and strength exercises result in a significant increase in bone densities from the second to fourth lumbar vertebrae in postmenopausal osteopenic women. Other benefits of physical exercise include improved balance and reduced risk of falls.

12. Bisphosphonates

In confirmed osteoporosis, this group of drugs belong to the first line of treatment and they are the most widely used and those with the most experience of use. The most commonly used are alendronic acid, 10 mg per day, or 70 mg per week, risedronic acid, 5 mg /day or 35 mg/week, ibrandonic acid 150 mg once a month, or zoldronic acid, 5 mg once a year intravenously.

Osteoporosis is caused by the decrease in the tissue that forms bone, both in the proteins that make up its matrix or structure and in the mineral salts of calcium it contains. As a consequence, the bone is less resistant and more fragile than normal [15].

Oral bisphosphonates have a relatively low absorption, and is recommended that food or liquids should not be ingested within 30 minutes of administration. They can cause side effects such as esophagitis and, rarely, jaw osteonecrosis. Zoledronic acid administered once a year intravenously does not present the problems of oral intolerance, but it frequently causes as a side- effect a picture of joint pain and fever that is not serious.

13. Teriparatide

It is an analog of human parathyroid hormone that is made up of a sequence of 34 amino acids, corresponding to the active fragment of the natural hormone. It is therefore a new bone-forming drug and is indicated in the treatment of osteoporosis.

It is used primarily in patients with established osteoporosis and a history of fractures, with particularly low bone mass, or with various risk factors for fractures. A daily injection of 20 micrograms is given subcutaneously. In some countries its use is only authorized if bisphosphonates have not been effective, or are contraindicated. Teriparatide is contraindicated in various circumstances, such as pregnancy, Paget's disease, hyperparathyroidism, and malignant tumors involving the bone [16].

14. Strontium Ranelate

It is an oral treatment alternative. It is effective in preventing vertebral fracture, but not hip fractures. It works by stimulating the proliferation of osteoblasts and also inhibits the proliferation of osteoclasts.

It is administered orally at a dose of 2 g daily. It does not have the side effects of bisphosphonates, as it does not cause gastric or esophageal symptoms. However, it has been shown to increase the risk of venous thromboembolism and can cause some serious dermatological reactions [17].

15. Hormone replacement therapy

15.1 Estrogens

Although it is known that estrogen treatment can be effective in stopping the loss of mineral content from bone in women after menopause, its administration as a treatment for osteoporosis is not currently recommended, due to the possibility of serious side effects and the existence of other safer alternatives. For this reason, estrogen therapy, as a hormonal treatment for menopause, is not recommended for the treatment of osteoporosis [18].

15.2 Testosterone

In men with testicular hypofunction, the administration of testosterone improves bone quantity and quality. However, there are no studies on its effects in reducing fractures or in men with normal testosterone levels [19].

15.3 Raloxifene

It is a selective estrogen receptor modulator. Drugs of this therapeutic group, bind to specific receptors on cells, simulating the activity of estrogens in certain tissues. Raloxifene acts on bone by decreasing osteoclast bone resorption and making vertebral fracture less likely. However, it is not effective in trying to reduce the incidence of hip fractures [20].

15.4 Denosumab

It is a drug that belongs to the group of biological agents, made up of monoclonal antibodies. In June 2010, its use was approved in the USA by the FDA to be used in the treatment of osteoporosis in post-menopausal women at high risk of fractures. Its mechanism of action is based on binding to a cellular receptor called RANKL, preventing its activation, which causes an inhibition in the formation of osteoclasts and their functionality. Osteoclasts are cells that are involved in the loss of bone mass and therefore favor the appearance of fractures [21, 22].

15.5 Prognosis

Patients with osteoporosis have an increased mortality rate, due to the greater likelihood of fractures occurring. The highest rate associated with osteoporosis is related to hip fractures, with an approximate mortality of 13.5% six months after they occur and 20–30% during the first year, which means that the risk of death, increases 2 to 10 times, higher than expected, in the population with similar characteristics. The causes of death are diverse and in many cases, they are not directly related to the presence of fractures.

The bad consequences of hip fractures are not limited to their hospital treatment, but to the deterioration of the quality of life, due to the residual disability that they entail. They can cause decreased mobility and the development of various complications, such as deep vein thrombosis, pulmonary embolism, and pneumonia.

At least 13% of the people who suffer them, need permanent help to be able to move. Vertebral fractures have less impact on mortality than hip fractures, but they can lead to thoracic and abdominal deformities, causing chronic pain that is difficult to control. Multiple vertebral fractures can lead to the appearance of significant lordosis and kyphosis of the spine, with the consequent increase in pressure on internal organs, which can decrease the respiratory capacity of affected subjects [23, 24].

Osteoporotic fractures are generally associated with a significant decrease in health-related quality of life [25].

Author details

Luis Rodrigo
Gastroenterology Department, University of Oviedo, Oviedo, Spain

*Address all correspondence to: lrodrigosaez@gmail.com

IntechOpen

References

[1] Elonheimo H, Lange R, Tolonen H, Kolossa-Gehring M. Environmental substances associated with osteoporosis. A Scoping Review. Int J Environ Res Public Health. 2021;18:73.

[2] Kim KT, Lee YS, Han I. The role of epigenomics in osteoporosis and osteoporotic vertebral fracture. Int J Mol Sci. 2020; 21: 9455.

[3] Burden AM, Tanaka Y, Xu L, Ha YC, McCloskey E, Cummings SR, Glüer CC. Osteoporosis case ascertainment strategies in European and Asian countries: A comparative review. Osteoporos Int. 2020 Dec. 10. doi : 10.1007/s00198-020-05756-8.

[4] Kanis JA, Harvey NC, Johansson H, Liu E, Vandenput L, Lorentzon M, Leslie WD, McCloskey EV. A decade of FRAX: How has it changed the management of osteoporosis?. Aging Clin Exp Res 2020: 32: 187-196.

[5] Chiodini I, Merlotti D, Falchetti A, Gennari L. Treatment options of glucocorticoid-induced osteoporosis. Expert Opin Pharmacother. 2020;21:721-732.

[6] Ding ZC, Zeng WN, Rong X, Liang ZM, Zhou ZK. Do patients with diabetes have an increased risk of impaired fracture healing? A systematic review and meta-analysis. ANZ J Surg. 2020; 90: 1259-1264.

[7] Mäkitie RE, Costantini A, Kämpe A, Alm JJ, Mäkitie O. New Insights Into Monogenic Causes of Osteoporosis. Front Endocrinol (Lausanne). 2019;10:70.

[8] Arima K, Mizukami S, Nishimura T, Tomita Y, Nakashima H, Abe Y, Aoyagi K. Epidemiology of the association between serum 25-hydroxyvitamin D levels and musculoskeletal conditions among elderly individuals: a literature review. J Physiol Anthropol. 2020;39:38.

[9] Veronese N, Kolk H, Maggi S. Epidemiology of Fragility Fractures and Social Impact. In: Orthogeriatrics: The Management of Older Patients with Fragility Fractures [Internet]. Cham (CH): Springer; 2021. Chapter 14.

[10] Warensjö Lemming E, Byberg L. Is a Healthy Diet Also Suitable for the Prevention of Fragility Fractures?. Nutrients. 2020;12:2642.

[11] Kennel KA, Sfeir JG, Drake MT. Optimizing DXA to Assess Skeletal Health: Key Concepts for Clinicians. J Clin Endocrinol Metab. 2020; 105:dgaa 632.

[12] Ciuffi S, Donati S, Marini F, Palmini G, Luzi E, Brandi ML. Circulating MicroRNAs as Novel Biomarkers for Osteoporosis and Fragility Fracture Risk: Is There a Use in Assessment Risk?. Int J Mol Sci. 2020;21:6927.

[13] Zhang X, Chen X, Xu Y, Yang J, Du L, Li K, Zhou Y. Milk consumption and multiple health outcomes: umbrella review of systematic reviews and meta-analyses in humans. Nutr Metab (Lond). 2021;18:7.

[14] Pinheiro MB, Oliveira J, Bauman A, Fairhall N, Kwok W, Sherrington C. Evidence on physical activity and osteoporosis prevention for people aged 65+ years: a systematic review to inform the WHO guidelines on physical activity and sedentary behaviour. Int J Behav Nutr Phys Act. 2020;17:150.

[15] Kuźnik A, Październiok-Holewa A, Jewula P, Kuźnik N. Bisphosphonates-much more than only drugs for bone diseases. Eur J Pharmacol. 2020;866:172773,

[16] Moon NH, Jang JH, Shin WC, Jung SJ. Effects of Teriparatide on Treatment Outcomes in Osteoporotic Hip and Pelvic Bone Fractures: Meta-analysis and Systematic Review of Randomized Controlled Trials. Hip Pelvis. 2020 ;32:182-191.

[17] Reginster JY, Brandi ML, Cannata-Andía J, Cooper C, Cortet B, Feron JM, Genant H, Palacios S, Ringe JD, Rizzoli R. The position of strontium ranelate in today's management of osteoporosis. Osteoporos Int. 2015;26:1667-1671.

[18] Mehta J, Kling JM, Manson JE. Risks, Benefits, and Treatment Modalities of Menopausal Hormone Therapy: Current Concepts. Front Endocrinol (Lausanne) 2021;12:564781.

[19] Chen JF, Lin PW, Tsai YR, Yang YC, Kang HY. Androgens and Androgen Receptor Actions on Bone Health and Disease: From Androgen Deficiency to Androgen Therapy. Cells. 2019; 8:1318.

[20] Pinkerton JV, Conner EA. Beyond estrogen: advances in tissue selective estrogen complexes and selective estrogen receptor modulators. Climacteric 2019;22:140-147.

[21] Anastasilakis AD, Makras P, Yavropoulou MP, Tabacco G, Naciu AM, Palermo A.J. Denosumab discontinuation and the rebound phenomenon: A narrative review. . Clin Med. 2021;10:152.

[22] Yasuda H. Discovery of the RANKL/RANK/OPG system. J Bone Miner Metab. 2021;39:2-11.

[23] Tanaka Y. Managing Osteoporosis and Joint Damage in Patients with Rheumatoid Arthritis: An Overview. J Clin Med. 2021;10:1241.

[24] Kim KT, Lee YS, Han I. The Role of Epigenomics in Osteoporosis and Osteoporotic Vertebral Fracture. Int J Mol Sci. 2020;21:9455.

[25] Coll PP, Phu S, Hajjar SH, Kirk B, Duque G, Taxel P. The prevention of osteoporosis and sarcopenia in older adults. J Am Geriatr Soc. 2021 Feb 23. Online ahead of print

Chapter 2

Glucocorticoid-Induced Osteoporosis

José Renan Vieira da Costa Júnior and Sérgio Luchini Batista

Abstract

The use of glucocorticoids (GC) in the medium and long term, causes several considerable side effects, being one of the main ones the reduction of bone mineral density (BMD). Prolonged corticosteroid therapy reduces BMD by up to 20% in trabecular bone and approximately 2–3% in cortical bone in the first year of use. This loss rate declines and stabilizes at approximately 2% in subsequent years. Therefore, there is a considerable increase in the incidence of pathological fractures, whether clinically symptomatic or asymptomatic (detected as a radiological finding), which varies between 30 and 50% of patients who use GC for more than three months. In view of the above, it is essential to prevent fractures and treat osteoporosis in patients using glucocorticoids for long periods (in particular, greater than or equal to 3 months), which may or may not be associated with clinical risk factors or previous fractures. The guidelines for the treatment and prevention of this comorbidity are well established for postmenopausal women and men over 50 years of age. However, for patients below this range, studies are still lacking.

Keywords: Osteoporosis, Glucocorticoids, Bone Fractures, Primary Prevention, Drug Therapy

1. Introduction

Glucocorticoids (GCs) are common medications in daily medical practice. About 0.5% and 1% of the populations in the United Kingdom and the United States use this drug class on an ongoing basis, respectively [1–17]. The use in the medium and long term, causes several considerable side effects, being one of the main ones the reduction of bone mineral density (BMD). Prolonged corticosteroid therapy reduces BMD by up to 20% in trabecular bone and approximately 2–3% in cortical bone in the first year of use. This loss rate declines and stabilizes at approximately 2% in subsequent years [1–9, 11–15, 17, 18].

Therefore, there is a considerable increase in the incidence of pathological fractures, whether clinically symptomatic or asymptomatic (detected as a radiological finding), which varies between 30 and 50% of patients who use GC for more than three months [1–31]. The fracture can be said to be pathological when it occurs with as little stress as possible and falls from one's own height, which would not cause fractures in healthy bones. The risk of fracture for a given BMD is greater in GC-induced osteoporosis (GIO) than senile or postmenopausal. In these last two, the stimulus for bone matrix synthesis is not affected [1–6, 11–15, 17, 26].

In view of the above, it is essential to prevent fractures and treat osteoporosis in patients using glucocorticoids for long periods (in particular, greater than or equal to 3 months), which may or may not be associated with clinical risk factors or previous fractures [1–31].

2. Pathogenesis

The side effects of corticosteroids on the bone system can occur indirectly or directly. Indirectly, corticosteroids increase urinary calcium excretion and vitamin D metabolism, reduce intestinal absorption of vitamin D, influence parathyroid hormone (PTH) secretion, reduce GH and IGF-1 levels and cause hypogonado-tropic hypogonadism (**Figure 1**). Directly, they act on osteoclasts by increasing the ligand of the nuclear factor activating receptor Kappa-B (RANK) and decreas-ing osteoprotegerin (OPG); on osteocytes causing apoptosis; and on osteoblasts inhibiting bone formation (**Figure 1**). The final effect is to reduce bone formation and stimulate its resorption, causing early bone loss and low bone mass in the long run. Trabecular bone is more prone to deleterious effects than cortical bone, with a more pronounced effect in the first year, especially in the first 6 months, and decays at a steady rate over the next few years. With chronic use, the stimulus to bone resorption is reduced and the suppression of bone formation becomes the dominant effect [2–7, 11–15, 17, 18, 26].

2.1 Increase in bone resorption

As in other tissues, glucocorticoids exert their effect from the genetic expres-sion of type 2 glucocorticoid cytoplasmic receptors. In adult bone, such receptors are found in pre-osteoblastic/stromal cells, the osteoblasts, which produce the bone matrix, but not in osteoclasts. GCs stimulate the proliferation of these cells by inhibiting the synthesis of osteoprotegerin, an inhibitor of the differentiation of hematopoietic cells of the macrophage lineage into osteoclasts and stimulating the production of RANK, which is necessary for osteoclastogenesis. High serum levels of GCs stimulate the synthesis of RANK ligands (RANKL), sustaining dif-ferentiation in osteoclasts and, consequently, bone matrix reabsorption (**Figure 2**). In addition, they reduce the production of androgens and estrogens, suppressing

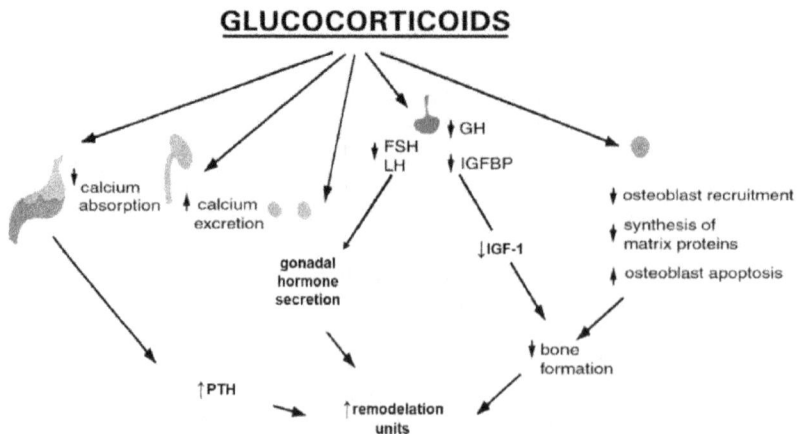

Figure 1.
Mechanisms of direct and indirect action of glucocorticoids on bone metabolism (Marcus et al., 2013, adapted) [11].

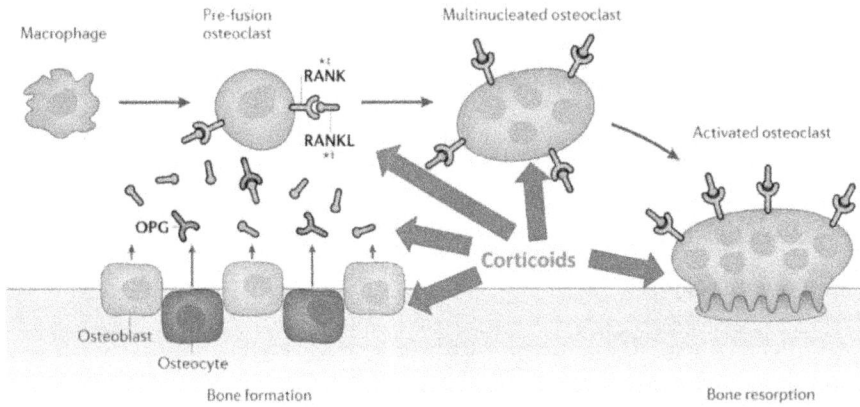

Figure 2.
Direct mechanisms of action of cortisol via the RANK/RANKL/OPG pathway (Richards et al., 2012, adapted) [26].

gonadotropin secretion by the adenohypophysis and consequent stimulus for bone resorption. GCs reduce intestinal calcium absorption, promoting antagonism to the action of vitamin D and by reducing the expression of calcium channels in the duodenum. They increase the excretion of calcium and reduce renal reabsorption. Both actions promote increased parathyroid hormone secretion and, consequently, bone resorption [2, 3, 5, 11–15, 17, 26].

2.2 Inhibition of bone formation

In GCs chronic use, the predominant effect will be the reduction of bone formation. This is generated by the direct reduction of osteoblastic proliferation and differentiation of precursors and stimulation of apoptosis of mature osteoblasts and osteocytes, increasing the risk of osteonecrosis. It changes the dynamics in the release of PTH, with reduced tonic secretion and increased pulses, inhibiting the anabolic action of this hormone. It also reduces the production of insulin-like growth factor (IGF-1) and testosterone. The reduction in bone formation is associated with a reduction in the rate of mineral apposition and can be documented by the low levels (serum and urinary) of biochemical markers of bone formation [2, 3, 5, 11–15, 17, 26].

3. Epidemiology and risk factors

The chronic use of GCs increases the risk of fractures, particularly in trabecular bones (in particular, vertebrae) and in the early phase of treatment, when the rate of bone loss is greatest. Its effect is greater in advancing age, dose and duration of treatment [2, 11–13, 17, 27]. A dose of 2.5–7.5 mg per day of prednisone (or equivalent), in less than 30 days, is enough to increase the risk of fractures. Below are patients with clinical risk factors for osteoporosis and pathological fractures [2, 11–13, 17, 27, 28]:
Major risk factors:

• History of previous fracture in adulthood;

• History of fracture in first-degree relatives;

- Current smoking;

- Low weight (BMI less than 18Kg/m^2);

- Concomitant diseases requiring chronic use of glucocorticoids (e.g., autoimmune inflammatory and pulmonary diseases, adrenal insufficiency).

Minor risk factors:

- Advanced age;

- Deficit of estrogen (e.g., menopause before the age of 45);

- Low calcium intake during life;

- Sedentary lifestyle;

- Alcoholism (3 or more doses of alcohol per day);

- Dementia (risk of falls).

4. Clinical findings

Generally, there are no clinical manifestations, except in the presence of fractures, in which there may be a stature reduction or local pain that worsens movement. The clinic will depend on the fractures involved. It is not uncommon to find asymptomatic fractures in imaging exams performed for other reasons. Patients with vertebral fracture (the main type involved), when symptomatic, present with low back pain that worsens when they get up, sit or cough. There is usually no history of associated trauma [7, 11–15].

5. Determining bone mineral density

The main standardized method for calculating bone mineral density is bone densitometry by dual-energy X-ray absorptiometry; (DXA). In addition, DXA can provide some additional information such as the presence of fractures through the VFA ("Vertebral Fracture Assessment") or changes in bone quality, through the TBS ("Trabecular Bone Score") [11–13, 15, 16, 21–25, 27, 29–31]. The World Health Organization (WHO) chooses this method, associated with the analysis of the results with the scores for the definition of Osteoporosis and Osteopenia. These scores are based on several studies with postmenopausal and white female patients (**Table 1**). There are two scores used [2, 4, 11–13, 15, 16, 21–25, 29, 30]:

- T-score: for postmenopausal women or men over 50 years old. Osteopenia is defined with a T-score between −1.1 and − 2.4 and osteoporosis less than or equal to −2.5.

- Z-score: for pre-menopausal women and men under 50 years old. If the score is less than or equal to −2.0, we should use the term "low bone mineral density adjusted for age and sex".

Criteria	Definitions
T-score	Number of SD above or below peak bone mass ("young normal") according to race or ethnicity
Z-score	Number of SD above or below age-matched bone mass according to gender and race or ethnicity
Normal	BMD T-score ≥ −1,0
Low bone mass (osteopenia)	BMD T-score between −1,1 and − 2,4
Osteoporosis	BMD T-score ≤ −2,5
Severe osteoporosis	BMD T-score ≤ −2,5 with one or more fragility fractures

BMD: bone mineral density; DXA: dual-energy X-ray absorptiometry; SD: standard-deviation; WHO: World Health Organization.

Table 1.
WHO definition of osteoporosis for postmenopausal women based on DXA measurements.

NOTE: The terms osteopenia and osteoporosis should be avoided in children, using the term "low bone mineral density for age and sex", if the Z-score is less than or equal to −2.0. The diagnosis of "osteoporosis" in children requires, associated with bone densitometry, at least 1 episode due to pathological fracture in a long bone in the lower limb or vertebra or 2 episodes in long bones in the upper limbs. Secondary causes of reduced bone mineral mass should be investigated in patients with a Z-score below −2.0. For this, use complementary exams such as 24-hour calciuria, which is usually increased in GIO [2, 11, 12, 15, 21–23, 27, 28].

Advanced bone mass measurement methods, including high resolution computed microtomography (micro-CT) and magnetic resonance imaging (micro-MR) allow for three-dimensional, non-invasive assessment of bone architecture. Although these methods help in the diagnosis of OIG, they are not used in medical practice, and their use is reserved only in clinical research [11, 12, 15, 23, 27, 28].

6. Approach to the patient on prolonged glucocorticoid therapy

Every adult patient using a dose greater than or equal to 2.5-5 mg per day for 3 months or more will benefit from osteoporosis prevention intervention. In children, candidates will be those who are using a dose greater than or equal to 0.16 mg/Kg/day or who have been submitted to at least 4 courses of pulses of glucocorticoids. Non-pharmacological measures and vitamin and calcium supplementation will be performed for all patients. For pharmacological therapy, there will be specific criteria [3, 5, 6, 11, 12, 15, 27, 28].

6.1 Candidates for pharmacological therapy

Determining factors, to high-risk fracture patients, who will benefit most from pharmacological therapy itself, are [3, 5, 6, 9–12, 15, 27, 28]:

- Patients with a previous diagnosis of osteoporosis (history of pathological fracture or T-score equal to or less than −2.5, calculated by bone densitometry).

- For patients without established osteoporosis, use tools that calculate the risk of pathological fracture, such as the fracture risk assessment tool (FRAX®).

6.2 FRAX®

FRAX® is a tool, created in 2008 by Dr. John Kanis of the University of Sheffield, that estimates the 10-year probability of hip fracture or combined major osteoporotic fractures (hip, vertebrae, shoulder or wrist) in untreated patients among 40–90 years, using bone mineral density of the femoral neck and associated clinical risk factors, including use of GCs [4, 8–13, 15, 16, 18, 21–25, 27, 29–31]. The percentage calculated by the tool must be corrected by the dose of GCs used. For example, for a patient using a prednisolone dose greater than 7.5 mg/day (or equivalent), the calculated risk of 15% for major osteoporotic fractures and 20% for hip fractures should be added to the calculated risk [2, 11–13, 15, 27].

In North America, the corrected calculations follow as possible results [2, 4, 8–13, 15, 16, 18, 21–25, 27, 29–31]:

- High risk: 10-year probability of a major combined osteoporotic or hip fracture greater than or equal to 20% and 3%, respectively.

- Moderate risk: 10-year probability of major combined osteoporotic or hip fracture between 10 and 19% and 1–3%, respectively.

- Low risk: 10-year probability of major combined osteoporotic or hip fracture less than 10% and 1%, respectively.

Patients can be at high risk for fractures even with FRAX® without being at high risk. For example, a patient with clinical factors for fractures and low lumbar bone mineral density, but with normal femoral neck bone density. This situation can occur especially in patients using GCs [11–13, 15, 27]. Trabecular bone score (TBS) could be used to access the bone quality and adjust risk fracture given by FRAX® [8–13, 15, 16, 18, 21–25, 29, 30]. Therefore, the treatment must be individualized between the patient and the attending physician [2, 5, 6, 11–13, 15, 27, 28].

6.3 For postmenopausal women and men over 50

Consider pharmacological therapy in patients with moderate to high risk [2, 5, 6, 11–13, 15, 27, 28]:

- Above patients with previous pathological fracture or bone densitometry with a T-score less than or equal to - 2.5 standard-deviations (SD), using any dose of glucocorticoid (prevention or treatment).

- High-risk men and postmenopausal women with a T-score between −1.1 and 2.4 SD using any dose of glucocorticoid. Perform the FRAX® calculation and assess high risk if total risk of osteoporotic and hip fracture greater than or equal to 20% and 3%, respectively.

- For postmenopausal women and men over 50 years old and with FRAX® with values lower than those reported above, we recommend starting pharmacological therapy if a dose of prednisone greater than or equal to 7.5 mg per day (or equivalent), for more than 3 months.

6.4 For pre-menopausal women and men under 50

The decision to start drug therapy must be individualized. In these individuals, the risk of fracture is not clearly defined and may differ from the risk of fracture in other populations using GCs. The FRAX® tool was not developed for this group of patients. It is suggested to evaluate treatment and, in case of hypogonadism, to associate hormone replacement therapy (to evaluate if there are any contraindications) [2, 11–13, 15, 27, 28].

Women should use highly effective contraceptives, given the lack of studies on the effects of drugs used in the treatment of GIO, especially bisphosphonates, on the fetus. Consider pharmacological treatment for the following groups of patients [2, 11–13, 15, 27, 28]:

- For pre-menopausal women and past pathological fractures;

- For pre-menopausal women without a past pathological fracture, but with accelerated bone loss (greater than or equal to 4% per year) or a Z-score less than −3.0, while receiving GCs with a prednisone dose greater than or equal to 7.5 mg per day (or equivalent) for 3 months or more).

- For men under 50 and with a past pathological fracture;

- Man under 50 years old with no past pathological fracture, but with accelerated bone loss (greater than or equal to 4% per year) or Z-score less than −3.0, while receiving GCs at a dose of prednisone greater than or equal to 7.5 mg per day (or equivalent) for 3 months or more;

- Men under 50 years old and pre-menopausal women and ingested more than 30 mg per day of prednisone (or equivalent) for more than 1 month.

7. Prevention and treatment

7.1 Non-pharmacological measures

The measures should be performed on all patients for whom treatment and prevention are indicated. Despite lacking studies on the reduction of fracture incidence, the American College of Rheumatology (ACR) defends the following [2, 5, 6, 10–13, 15, 27, 28]:

- Dose of glucocorticoid should be the lowest possible for resolution of the target disease;

- When possible, topical therapy (ointments, inhaled corticosteroids) will be preferable if compared with oral and intravenous corticosteroids (these have systemic effects), according to the associated pathology to be treated;

- Performing physical exercises with moderate muscle impact to reduce bone loss;

- Cessation or avoiding smoking;

- Limit alcohol intake to 3 doses a day or stop using it;

- Measures to prevent falls (especially in patients with dementia and the elderly).

7.2 Calcium and vitamin D supplementation

GCs induce a negative balance by reducing intestinal calcium absorption and increasing their urinary excretion. Thus, for all patients using corticosteroids for 3 months or more, it is recommended to keep calcium intake between 600 and 1200 mg of elemental calcium per day and vitamin D between 400 and 800 IU/ day [2, 5, 6, 10–13, 15, 27, 28]. These doses can be in the diet or supplementation. Maintain serum vitamin D levels greater than or equal to 20 ng/dL. Another measure would be the low sodium diet, aiming to reduce calciuria and, if necessary, to introduce thiazide diuretics [2, 11, 12, 15, 27, 28].

Such measures, despite reducing the rate of bone density loss, are not sufficient to prevent bone mass loss and pathological fractures in patients using high doses of GCs. In some cases, pharmacological therapy is necessary, with the use of active metabolites of vitamin D (such as calcitriol and alpha-calcidiol), which have greater action. Calcitriol (0.25 mcg per day) associated with calcium has a greater protective effect against vertebral fractures than the isolated use of calcium in patients using GCs. However, active vitamin D metabolites are at increased risk of hypercalcemia and hypercalciuria. In addition, some studies demonstrate less effectiveness of these when compared to medications already on the market, such as bisphosphonates, for example [2, 10–12, 15, 27, 28].

7.3 Hormonal replacement in hypogonadism

In patients with hypogonadism, GCs can reduce the release of gonadotropins and, consequently, estrogens and androgens. In this group, as long as there are no contraindications, hormone replacement is indicated. For women in menopause, who are hypogonadic and using GC, replacement of estrogen/progestin form is indicated. Oral contraceptives can be started until treatment with corticosteroids ceases. If contraindications to oral contraceptives (migraine with aura, important side effects), standard doses of estradiol and progesterone can be used. In a patient with normal ovarian function, hormone replacement is not indicated [11–13, 15, 27, 28].

7.4 Pharmacological treatment - therapy of choice

In men and postmenopausal women, bisphosphonates are the class of choice. Alendronate and risendronate are preferable because they have larger studies and better efficacy in them. For patients with drug intolerance, difficulty with dosage or adherence, intravenous zoledronic acid (zoledronate) is preferable [2, 5, 6, 9–13, 15, 27, 28].

Parathormone or analogues such as teriparatide are indicated for patients with severe osteoporosis: T-score less than −3.5 SD without fractures or below −2.5 SD and history of pathological fracture preferable [2, 5, 6, 9–13, 15, 27, 28].

Teriparatide is an option if there is an intolerance to bisphosphonates or if there is a fracture after 1 year of treatment with 1st line drugs. Denosumab is a therapeutic alternative for those at high risk of fracture. However, there is a high incidence of vertebral fractures after discontinuing medication (start only if there are no alternatives for further treatment) [2, 5, 6, 9–13, 15, 19, 27, 28].

In premenopausal women who do not need hormone replacement, bisphosphonates are the class of choice. Teriparatide is second line, as long as there is radiological evidence of epiphyseal fusion of the long bones. Denosumab may also be an option in patients at high risk for fractures preferable [2, 5, 6, 9–13, 15, 19, 27, 28].

In addition to the new ACR guidelines, published in 2017, we also have the guidelines of the International Osteoporosis Foundation - European Calcified Tissue Society (IOF-ECTS), published in 2012, illustrated below (**Figures 3** and **4**) [2, 9, 10].

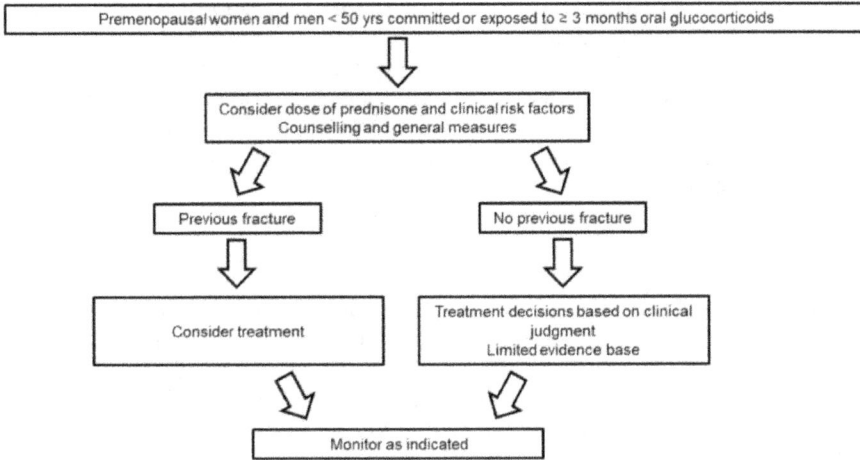

Figure 3.
Guidelines for the treatment of premenopausal women and men aged less than 50 from the joint international osteoporosis foundation (IOF) - European calcified tissue society (ECTS) glucocorticoid-induced osteoporosis (GIO) [9, 10].

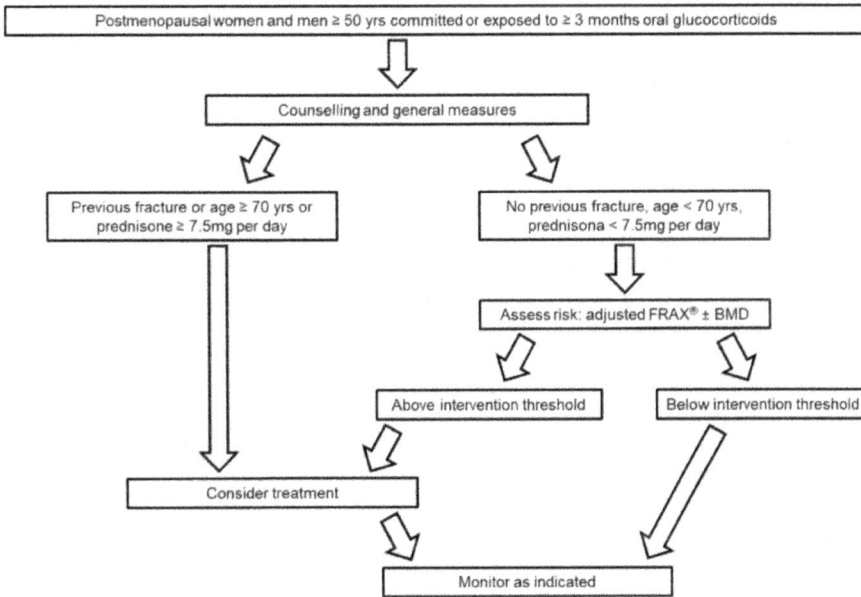

Figure 4.
Guidelines for the treatment of postmenopausal women and men aged 50 and over from the joint international osteoporosis foundation (IOF) - European calcified tissue society (ECTS) glucocorticoid-induced osteoporosis (GIO) [9, 10].

7.4.1 Effectiveness of pharmacological treatment

7.4.1.1 Bisphosphonates

Class responsible for increasing the half-life of osteoblasts. For a long time, it was believed that the protective effect of this class was due to its pro-apoptotic effect of osteoclasts. However, GC can inhibit this effect on osteoclasts, reducing drug efficacy [2, 9–13, 15, 27, 28].

For women and men who are candidates for pharmacological therapy, these are the first line of prevention and treatment of bone loss induced by glucocorticoids. Especially alendronate and risendronate. A meta-analysis of 27 clinical trials showed a significant reduction in bone mass and structure improvement and a consequent reduction in fractures in the lumbar vertebrae and femoral neck. The reduction of non-vertebral fractures was not statistically significant [2, 9–13, 15, 27, 28].

There is not enough data to indicate the use of medications in pregnant women. Further studies are needed [2, 11–13, 15, 27, 28]. Below are the main representatives of the class:

Alendronate: Studies have shown an improvement in global bone density and a reduction in hip and femur fractures. There is no evidence of improvement in vertebra fractures. The protective effect was maintained for 2 years. Standard dose: 5-10 mg, orally, daily or 35-70 mg, orally, weekly [2, 9–13, 15, 27, 28].

Risendronate: studies have shown a reduction in the incidence of lumbar vertebral and femoral neck fractures. Standard dose: 5 mg, orally, daily or 35 mg, orally, weekly [2, 9–13, 15, 27, 28].

Zoledronic acid (zoledronate): studies have shown a reduction in vertebral fractures, especially in high-risk patients. Standard dose: 5 mg, intravenous, annual. In the first three days after application, adverse effects such as arthralgia, fever, flu-like symptoms and, more rarely, hypocalcemia, which are more common in the first dose of this medication, may reduce the risk in subsequent doses [2, 9–13, 15, 27, 28].

Other bisphosphonates: pamidronate (oral and intravenous) can reduce the rate of bone loss induced by GC, but it has been replaced by zoledronic acid. Regarding ibandronate, studies for its routine use in GIO are lacking [11–13, 15, 27, 28].

7.4.1.2 Parathormone (PTH)

PTH stimulates bone formation as well as its resorption and its intermittent administration stimulates bone formation more than resorption [2, 9–13, 15, 27, 28]. In randomized studies, PTH showed a greater reduction in vertebral and femoral neck fractures than alendronate. The rate of non-vertebral fractures was similar with both medications [2, 11–13, 15, 27, 28].

Despite its great efficacy, it is not the first choice for treatment or prevention of osteoporosis induced by glucocorticoids, given its cost, subcutaneous administration and availability of other medications [2, 11–13, 15, 27, 28]. Indicated for treatment in postmenopausal women and men aged 50 or over in the following situations [2, 11–13, 15, 27, 28]:

- Severe osteoporosis (T-score less than or equal to −3.5 without fractures or previous episode of pathological fracture and T-score less than or equal to −2.5) before starting glucocorticoids.

- Osteoporosis (T-score less than −2.5) in patients who do not tolerate the use of bisphosphonates or who are contraindicated to oral bisphosphonates due to achalasia, esophageal scleroderma or esophageal stenosis, for example.

- Failure of other therapies: fracture with loss of bone density even with prevention or treatment.

Teriparatide (exogenous PTH) is an option for women of childbearing age as long as the epiphyses show radiological signs of fusion, a history of pathological fractures or accelerated bone loss (equal to or greater than 4% per year), while using glucocorticoids (minimum 7.5 mg per day of prednisone for 3 months or more) and there is no need for hormone replacement therapy. Its use is not recommended for more than 2 years due to the potential risk of osteosarcoma. For patients who receive the medication, but remain at high risk for fractures, it is recommended to start bisphosphonates soon after its completion. Standard dose: 20mcg per day, subcutaneous [2, 11–13, 15, 27, 28].

Abaloparatide (synthetic analogue of PTH-related protein), although promising, still does not have enough studies to indicate its routine use in GIO [11–13, 15, 27, 28].

7.4.1.3 Other pharmacological therapies

Denosumab: monoclonal antibody against RANKL, acts by inhibiting osteoclast formation and differentiation and re3ducing bone resorption, with a consequent increase in bone mineral density and reducing the risk of vertebral fracture. Used in postmenopausal women and men undergoing androgen deprivation treatment for prostate cancer. After discontinuation of use, the risk of vertebral fractures increases considerably. Analyze with the patient, treatment alternatives (usually bisphosphonates) after their removal to the segment. Standard dose: 60 mg, subcutaneous, every 6 months [2, 9–13, 15, 19, 27, 28].

Romosozumab: a potent anabolic anti-sclerostin antibody that could be considered as a substitute for PTH analogs. However, it lacks studies for its indication in GIO [4 18, 19, 21, 24, 25, 28].

Calcitonin: widely used in the past, but not very effective, it is currently not recommended for use because there are better treatment alternatives [2, 11–13, 15, 27, 28].

8. Monitoring

The guidelines guide the monitoring of BMD for the treatment segment. There is no consensus as to the frequency and period for measuring bone mineral density, but it is suggested that [2, 9–13, 15, 27, 28]:

- If density of bone mass stable or rising: every 6 months in the first year and every 1–2 years in subsequent years, this interval can be increased for every 2–3 years;

- If bone mass density is decreasing or a new fracture is still being treated: investigate poor adherence to treatment, gastrointestinal absorption disorder, association of another disease with skeletal involvement, change to injectable medication in case of failure with oral treatment.

9. Conclusion

Glucocorticoids are medications widely used in continuous treatments in a significant portion of the world population. Given this, its continued use has considerable side effects, especially OIG. The guidelines for the treatment and prevention of this comorbidity are well established for postmenopausal women and men over 50 years of age. However, for patients below this range, studies are still lacking [2, 11–13, 15, 27, 28].

Author details

José Renan Vieira da Costa Júnior[1] and Sérgio Luchini Batista[2*]

1 Physician at the Internal Medicine Residency Program at Santa Casa de Misericórdia de Ribeirão Preto, Ribeirão Preto, SP, Brazil

2 Full Professor at Medicine Course at Centro Universitário Barão de Mauá, Ribeirão Preto, SP, Brazil

*Address all correspondence to: luchinifmrp@gmail.com

IntechOpen

References

[1] Adler RA. Glucocorticoid-Induced Osteoporosis: Management Challenges in Older Patients. J Clin Densitom 2019. DOI: 10.1016/j.jocd.2018.03.004.

[2] Buckley L, et al. 2017 American College of Rheumatology Guideline for the Prevention and Treatment of Glucocorticoid-Induced Osteoporosis. Arthritis & Rheumatology, DOI: 10.1002/art.40137.

[3] Canalis E, Mazziotti G, Giustina A, Bilezikian JP. Glucocorticoid-induced osteoporosis: pathophysiology and therapy. Osteoporos Int. 2007. DOI: 10.1007/s00198-007-0394-0.

[4] Carter M. Prevention of Glucocorticoid-Induced Osteoporosis: Clinical audit to evaluate the implementation of National Osteoporosis Guideline Group 2017 guidelines in a primary care setting. J Clin Densitom. 2019. DOI: 10.1016/j.jocd.2018.03.009.

[5] Chotiyarnwong P, McCloskey EV. Pathogenesis of glucocorticoid-induced osteoporosis and options for treatment. Nat Rev Endocrinol. 2020. DOI: 10.1038/s41574-020-0341-0.

[6] Compston J. Glucocorticoid-induced osteoporosis: an update. Endocrine. 2018. DOI: 10.1007/s12020-018-1588-2.

[7] Lane NE. Glucocorticoid-Induced Osteoporosis: New Insights into the Pathophysiology and Treatments. Curr Osteoporos Rep. 2019. DOI: 10.1007/s11914-019-00498-x.

[8] Leib ES, Saag KG, Adachi JD, Geusens PP, Binkley N, McCloskey EV, Hans DB. FRAX(®) Position Development Conference Members. Official Positions for FRAX(®) clinical regarding glucocorticoids: the impact of the use of glucocorticoids on the estimate by FRAX(®) of the 10 year risk of fracture from Joint Official Positions Development Conference of the International Society for Clinical Densitometry and International Osteoporosis Foundation on FRAX(®). J Clin Densitom. 2011. DOI: 10.1016/j.jocd.2011.05.014.

[9] Lekamwasam S, Adachi JD, Agnusdei D, Bilezikian J, Boonen S, Borgström F, Cooper C, Diez Perez A, Eastell R, Hofbauer LC, Kanis JA, Langdahl BL, Lesnyak O, Lorenc R, McCloskey E, Messina OD, Napoli N, Obermayer-Pietsch B, Ralston SH, Sambrook PN, Silverman S, Sosa M, Stepan J, Suppan G, Wahl DA, Compston JE. Joint IOF-ECTS GIO Guidelines Working Group. A framework for the development of guidelines for the management of glucocorticoid-induced osteoporosis. Osteoporos Int. 2012. DOI: 10.1007/s00198-012-1958-1.

[10] Lekamwasam, S. et al. An appendix the 2012 IOF–ECTS guidelines for the management of glucocorticoid-induced osteoporosis. Archive Osteoporosis, 2012. DOI: 10.1007/s11657-012-0070-7.

[11] Marcus R, Feldman D, Dempster DW, Luckey M, Cauley J, editors. Osteoporosis. 4th ed, Waltham: Elsevier. 2013. 2116p. DOI: 10.1002/9780124158535.

[12] Pereira RMR, et al. Guidelines for the prevention and treatment of glucocorticoid-induced osteoporosis. Brazilian journal of Rheumatology, 2012 [Internet]. Available from: https://pubmed.ncbi.nlm.nih.gov/22885424/ [Accessed: 2021/03/01].

[13] Pereira RMR. Glucocorticoid-induced osteoporosis: prevention and treatment. Project Guidelines [Internet]. 2011. Available from: saudedireta.com.br/docsupload/

1331159316osteoporose_induzida_por_glicocorticoide.pdf [Accessed: 2021-03-01].

[14] Rosen HN. Clinical features and evaluation of glucocorticoid-induced osteoporosis. UpToDate [Internet]. 2021; Available from: https://www.uptodate.com/contents/clinical-features-and-evaluation-of-glucocorticoid-induced-osteoporosis?search=osteoporosis%20glucocorticoid&source=search_result&selectedTitle=2~150&usage_type=default&display_rank=2 [Accessed: 2021-03-01].

[15] Shoback D. Osteoporosis & Glucocorticoid-induced Osteoporosis. In: Imboden JB, Hellmann DB, Stone JH, et al. CURRENT diagnosis & tratment Rheumatology. 3rd ed. Chicago: McGrawHill; 2013. p. 433-451. DOI: 10.1002/9780071638067.ch58.

[16] Wallace B, Saag KG, Curtis JR, Waljee AK. Just the FRAX: Management of Glucocorticoid-Induced Osteoporosis. Gastroenterology. 2018. DOI: 10.1053/j.gastro.2018.01.016.

[17] Wang L, Heckmann BL, Yang X, Long H. Osteoblast autophagy in glucocorticoid-induced osteoporosis. J Cell Physiol. 2019. DOI: 10.1002/jcp.27335.

[18] Kanis JA, Johnell O, Oden A, Johansson H, McCloskey E. FRAX and the assessment of fracture probability in men and women from the UK. Osteoporos Int. 2008. DOI: 10.1007/s00198-007-0543-5.

[19] Benlidayi IC. Denosumab in the treatment of glucocorticoid-induced osteoporosis. Rheumatol Int. 2018. DOI: 10.1007/s00296-018-4106-1.

[20] Buckley L, Humphrey MB. Glucocorticoid-Induced Osteoporosis. N Engl J Med. DOI: 10.1056/NEJMcp1800214.

[21] Hans, D. et al. Bone microarchitecture assessed by TBS predicts osteoporotic fractures independent of bone density: the Manitoba study. J Bone Miner Res. 2011. DOI: 10.1002/jbmr.499.

[22] Harvey NC, et al. Trabecular bone score (TBS) as a new complementary approach for osteoporosis evaluation in clinical practice. Bone, 2015. DOI: 10.1016/j.bone.2015.05.016.

[23] Hatipoglu HG, et al. Quantitative and diffusion MR imaging as a new method to assess osteoporosis. AJNR Am J Neuroradiol. 2007. DOI: 10.3174/ajnr.A0704.

[24] Lewiecki E.M. Osteoporotic fracture risk assessment. UpToDate [Internet]. 2021. Available from: https://www.uptodate.com/contents/osteoporotic-fracture-risk-assessment?sectionName=CLINICAL%20RISK%20FACTOR%20ASSESSMENT&topicRef=2032&anchor=H17&source=see_link#H17 [Accessed: 2021-03-01].

[25] Rajan R, Cherian KE, Kapoor N, Paul TV. Trabecular Bone Score-An Emerging Tool in the Management of Osteoporosis. Indian J Endocrinol Metab. 2020. DOI: 10.4103/ijem.IJEM_147_20.

[26] Richards JB, Zheng HF, Spector TD. Genetics of osteoporosis from genome-wide association studies: advances and challenges. In: (Ed.). Nat Rev Genet. England, v.13, 2012. PMID: 22805710

[27] Rosen HN, Drezner MK. Overview of the management of osteoporosis in postmenopausal women. UpToDate [Internet]. 2021; Available from: https://www.uptodate.com/contents/overview-of-the-management-of-osteoporosis-in-postmenopausal-women?search=osteoporosis&source=search_result&selectedTitle=1~150&usage_type=default&display_rank=1 [Accessed: 2021-03-01].

[28] Rosen HN. Prevention and treatment of glucocorticoid-induced osteoporosis. UpToDate [Internet]. 2021; Available from: https://www.uptodate.com/contents/prevention-and-treatment-of-glucocorticoid-induced-osteoporosis?search=glucocorticoid%20osteoporosis&source=search_result&selectedTitle=1~150&usage_type=default&display_rank=1 [Accessed: 2021-03-01].

[29] Sandru F, Carsote M, Dumitrascu MC, Albu SE, Valea A. Glucocorticoids and Trabecular Bone Score. J Med Life. 2020. DOI: 10.25122/jml-2019-0131.

[30] Shevroja E, Lamy O, Kohlmeier L, Koromani F, Rivadeneira F, Hans D. Use of Trabecular Bone Score (TBS) as a Complementary Approach to Dual-energy X-ray Absorptiometry (DXA) for Fracture Risk Assessment in Clinical Practice. J Clin Densitom. 2017. DOI: 10.1016/j.jocd.2017.06.019.

[31] Warzecha M, Czerwiński E, Amarowicz J, Berwecka M. Trabecular Bone Score (TBS) in Clinical Practice - Rewiev. Ortop Traumatol Rehabil. 2018. DOI: 10.5604/01.3001.0012.7281.

Chapter 3

Osteoporosis and Dietary Inflammatory Index

Olga Cvijanović Peloza, Sandra Pavičić Žeželj,
Gordana Kenđel Jovanović, Ivana Pavičić,
Ana Terezija Jerbić Radetić, Sanja Zoričić Cvek,
Jasna Lulić Drenjak, Gordana Starčević Klasan,
Ariana Fužinac Smojver and Juraj Arbanas

Abstract

Healthy bones are constantly being renewed and proper nutrition is an important factor in this process. Anti-inflammatory diet is designed to improve health and prevent the occurrence and development of chronic diseases associated with inadequate diet. Proper nutrition is based on the anti-inflammatory pyramid and changes in poor eating habits are the long-term strategy for preventing inflammation and chronic diseases. Inflammatory factors from food may play a role in the development of osteoporosis and an anti-inflammatory diet may be a way to control and reduce long-term inflammation and prevent bone loss. Pro-inflammatory cytokines from the fat tissue, through activation of the RANKL/RANK/OPG system could intervene with bone metabolism in a way of increased bone loss. Therefore the special attention need to be given to obese patients due to twofold risk, one related to pro-inflammatory cytokines release and the other related to the deprivation of the vitamin D in the fat tissue.

Keywords: chronic diseases, cytokines, dietary inflammatory index, obesity, osteoporosis

1. Introduction

Along with water and oxygen, food is the basis of life. The food contains essential compounds, and their lack leads to imbalance, affects the metabolism and functioning of organic systems, creating a prerequisite for diseases [1]. Adequate nutrition is one of the crucial factors in maintaining good health in adulthood. It also forms the basis of proper growth and development of children and adolescents [2].

The main guidelines for improving nutrition are listed in the National Food Policies. Similarly to existing policies, the Croatian Food Policy, states that proper nutrition is one that:

- establishes a balance between energy ingested by food and energy consumed;

- allows proper distribution between carbohydrates, fats and proteins;

- ensures a sufficient amount of minerals;

- ensures sufficient intake of vitamins;

- provides the body's needs for water [3].

According to data available from the World Health Organization, it is important to recognize the dangers arising from excessive food consumption and the danger of insufficient energy intake of some nutrients. Hundreds of millions of people suffer from diseases that are the result of an unbalanced diet or consuming excessive amounts of food. There is increasing data that diet rich in lipids, rather saturated fatty acids than unsaturated, high intake of sugar and sodium, but lower intake of micronutrients and complex carbohydrates leads to an increase in cardiovascular diseases, obesity, diabetes, osteoporosis, and cancer [4].

Available data that refers to the science of nutrition, suggest two major directions in history. Firstly, energy intake and nutritional needs were investigated, while nowadays, research is focused on nutrients that have a positive impact on human health and the impact of diet on gene expression [5].

Many nutrients have been linked to bone health, including some like dairy, fish, vegetables and soy which can improve it, while unbalanced and salty diet can influence it negatively. Calcium is the most abundant mineral in the body, 1.5-2% of total body weight is mostly found in bones and teeth, about 99% and 1% is found in extracellular fluid and soft tissues. Calcium plays a role in regulating normal muscle and nerve irritability, regulates cell membrane permeability to sodium and participates in blood coagulation. Calcium ingested with food is absorbed by 10-30%. There is an increased need for calcium in pregnancy and lactation [6]. Milk and dairy products are the best sources of calcium, but it can also be found in some types of green leafy vegetables, fish, meat, and grains [7]. The recommended daily intake of calcium in Croatia is 800 mg [8].

Phosphorus is also linked to bone health. Phosphorous and calcium are major constituents of the hydroxyapatite [9]. Recommended daily intake of phosphorus is 700 mg/day [9]. Foods rich in phosphorus are fish, meat, cereals and carbonated beverages [10].

Vitamin D plays a leading role in bone health. It is a fat-soluble vitamin and needs bile salts for its absorption [6]. The metabolism of phosphorus and calcium affects the physiological role of vitamin D, as it conditions their resorption and deposition in bone tissue. Vitamin D deficiency in the body causes rickets in children, and osteomyelitis in adults [6]. Vitamin D is found in eggs, liver, fish oil and butter. Food is poor in vitamin D, so it is necessary to expose the skin to UV radiation.

Proteins of animal or vegetable origin are important part of the diet of children and adults. The recommended daily protein intake is 0.8 g/kg per day and is not sufficient for the elderly [11, 12]. Proteins are needed for the collagen synthesis in bone and have a positive effect on bone health especially in the elderly when protein-energy malnutrition leads to an increased risk of fractures [11].

In addition to macronutrient proteins, fats additionally affect bone. Fats area unit outlined as organic compounds found in foods of animal and plant origin. The role of fats within the body is multiple: additionally to carbohydrates, they are the most supply of energy, change the perform of nerve impulses, regulate temperature, and area unit carriers of fat-soluble vitamins. The counseled daily fat intake ought to be a minimum of 15% of the overall daily energy intake (WHO) [6]. Diet wealthy in saturated fatty acids and lack of physical activity will result in blubber. Fat tissue produces adipokines, which are pleiotropic molecules that not solely regulate food intake and energy metabolism however are concerned within the complicated interactions between fat tissue and bone [13, 14]. Some investigations imply that cytokines of fat tissue intervene with bone metabolism. General inflammation, a key element within the pathological process of metabolic syndrome, could negatively influence bone health [15].

The anti-inflammatory diet is similar to the Mediterranean diet, designed to improve health and to prevent the occurrence and development of chronic diseases associated with an inadequate diet. Excessive consumption of certain foods, especially industrially processed, stress, insufficient physical activity and too much adipose tissue cause low-grade chronic inflammation, which can precipitate cardiovascular disease, insulin resistance, type II diabetes, arthritis, neurological diseases, thyroid disease, carcinomas and some mental diseases. An anti-inflammatory diet does not necessarily mean a major change to the usual diet, it may contain local, common foods, but it is of utmost importance to avoid food with a high risk for diseases. On the other hand, an anti-inflammatory diet provides a certain ratio of nutrients that regulate energy consumption in a better way, acts on satiety and consumes less energy.

It is important to note that this diet is rich in many nutrients that balance health and prevent the onset and development of various chronic diseases.

In addition to the usual foods that make up the Mediterranean diet, the basis of the anti-inflammatory diet is vegetables that grow above ground - cabbage, broccoli, cauliflower, kale, Brussels sprouts, spinach, chicory, chard, kale, eggplant, olives, beans, artichokes, asparagus, zucchini, lettuce, endive, dill, chicory, rocket, cucumbers, tomatoes, peppers, fennel, celery, pumpkin, onions, spring onions, shallots, garlic, leeks.

Of the fruits, these are avocado, lemon, and spices such as ginger, turmeric with pure herbs that have a special role - parsley leaf, thyme, oregano, basil, rosemary, sage, cinnamon, cumin, clove, mint, lavender, anise, and fennel. Of the oils, cold-pressed oils are recommended - olive, pumpkin, flaxseed, and less often hemp and coconut [16].

2. Osteoporosis and dietary inflammatory index

Postmenopausal osteoporosis is characterized by rapid bone loss, especially in during the first 5 years of the menopause. Clinical symptoms of osteoporosis are usually not present, which is why it is called silent disease. Decrease in estrogen levels trigger numerous changes in bone metabolism which result in bone mass loss and bone quality disorders. They firstly alter trabecular bone and subsequently cortical frame, all together leading to fracture of single bones. Fractures can occur in any bone, but mostly affect hip, vertebrae of the spine, and wrist [17].

In clinical practice, there are several approaches in diagnosing osteoporosis, and they can all fall into two categories:

- Clinical assessment of risk factors for osteoporosis

- Determination of bone mineral density (BMD)

The technique most commonly used by physicians to make a quantitative diagnosis of osteoporosis is to measure bone mineral density by dual-energy X-ray absorptiometry - DEXA. The advantage of this technique is simple and quick application, which enables BMD values to be available to the physician in a short period of time. Usually, BMD is measured in the places that are most susceptible to fractures (hip, spine and forearm). Based on bone mineral density values, the World Health Organization has defined indicators for the diagnosis of osteoporosis in menopausal women. Thus, osteoporosis can be diagnosed in women whose BMD values are 2.5 and more standard deviations (SD) lower than the average peak bone mass values that apply to young, healthy, white women (standard). By comparing the measured values of BMD and standards (peak bone mass), the T coefficient is obtained. The Z coefficient represents the deviation of the measured value of BMD from the average bone mass of persons of the same age, expressed in standard deviations. Values of T coefficient of -2.5 and less, and Z coefficient of -1 and less, speak in favor of osteoporosis. Values of T > 1 indicate increased bone mass; values of T coefficient between -1 and -2 indicate osteopenia and those values of T coefficient between -1 and -2.5 indicate normal bone mass [17]. Numerous prospective studies have given bone mineral density results that have shown a good association with the occurrence of fractures in subjects (R2 = 0.4 - 0.9). In a study conducted by Marshall et al. on 90,000 women, more than 2,000 of whom had fractures, it was shown, that decrease in BMD of 1 SD for a given age, is associated with the risk of one to one and a half bone fractures [17]. Referring to the results of Marshall et al., BMD values have increasingly been used in clinical practice to assess the risk of bone fractures. However, there are a number of limiting circumstances that do not allow the notion of BMD as a surrogate in the assessment of bone strength and bone biomechanical abilities. Interpretation of BMD values is sometimes illogical and cannot be used in fracture risk assessment. This is supported by the finding of 50% of women who had a fracture, and whose BMD values measured on the spine and hip were above the -2.5 SD threshold to be able to diagnose osteoporosis at all. Another limitation relates to faults that occur during scanning, so that poor patient position or changes in patient orientation in serial images give inaccurate BMD values or values that are often difficult to interpret [18]. Risk factors for bone fractures include excessive alcohol consumption, female gender, positive fracture in medical history, female hip fracture, oral glucocorticoid use, lack of physical activity and nutritional factors [18, 19]. Lifestyle factors which are the most investigated in relation to bone health are nutrition and physical activity. Recent Meta-Analyses showed that exercises can significantly improve trabecular volumetric BMD values measured on tibia and can increase lumbar spine and femoral neck BMD, in post-menopausal women [19]. Mechanical strain activates osteocytes, which initiate bone remodeling resulting in repair of bone tissue damaged by microcracks. On the opposite, bone damage or long-term immobilization results in osteocyte apoptosis and increased osteoclastogenesis.

Low values of body mass index are also associated with the risk of bone fractures as well as low values of bone mineral density [18]. When for some reason it is not possible to determine bone mineral density values, then the body mass index provides useful data to assess fracture risk. It can be said that the above risk factors are not in themselves sufficient in the assessment of fracture risk or in the assessment of bone mineral density values. However, risk factors are useful as a complement to the densitometry finding in the clinical interpretation of fracture risk. The intensity of bone remodeling can be assessed by determining the values of biochemical markers in serum and urine [20].

Under physiological conditions, bone remodeling maintains the bone mass that the body needs not only for metabolic needs, but also to perform important biomechanical functions.

Higher intensity of bone resorption leads to a negative balance of bone remodeling which affects the change of structural and material properties of bone.

Bone resorption markers include tartrate-resistant acid phosphatase (TRAP) and type I collagen cleavage products such as C-terminal telopeptide (CTx),

N-terminal telopeptide (NTx), and deoxypyridinoline. Bone-forming markers include bone-specific alkaline phosphatase (bALP), osteocalcin and residuals that are released by the action of lysine on the procollagen molecule [20]. A large number of investigations which have taken inflammatory etiology of osteoporosis into consideration, have measured experimentally and also in patients the levels of the receptor activator of nuclear factor κB (RANK), its functional ligand (sRANKL) and decoy receptor to RANKL, osteoprotegerin (OPG). sRANKL is a member of the TNF-α family of the cytokines and induces maturation, differentiation and activity of osteoclasts in direct manner or indirectly, as result of macrophage-colony stimulating factor stimulation. Estrogen related bone loss, which is pronounced in the first 5 years of the menopause can be also related to RANKL activation. Care should be taken in determining the value of bone markers so that the results obtained are not misinterpreted [21, 22] .

To relate research with dietary inflammatory potential and its effect on human health, scientists have developed and validated the "Dietary Inflammatory Index - DII" [23]. DII has been shown to be statistically significantly associated with inflammatory biomarkers, particularly IL-6, TNF-α, hs-CRP, and with the combined score of inflammatory biomarkers [24]. DII is an index for assessment of an individual's dietary inflammatory ability, designed on 1943 scientific papers, and is composed of 45 nutritional parameters, which are rated according to pro-inflammatory or anti-inflammatory effect [23] (**Table 1**). It is based on results published in the scientific literature and then standardized with global intake values for all dietary parameters included in the DII index. (Parameter that has a pro-inflammatory effect is scored with +1, while parameter with anti-inflammatory effect with -1 and with 0 parameters without effect. The DII index is increasingly used to assess the association of the inflammatory potential of the diet with various inflammatory chronic diseases [25], cardiovascular disease [25], carcinomas [26–33], premature death as a result of chronic non-communicable diseases [25], asthma [34] and depression and anxiety [35, 36] (**Table 2**). The biggest potential of the DII index is in the selection of anti-inflammatory food, and control over inflammatory diseases.

Nutrient	Inflammation effective score[*]	World average daily intake	Nutrient	Inflammation effective score[*]	World average daily intake
Curcuma	-0,785	533 mg	Saturated fats	0,373	28,6 g
Isoflavonoids	-0,593	1,20 mg	Total fats	0,298	71,4 g
Beta carotene	-0,584	3718 mcg	Trans fats	0,229	3,15 g
Green/black tea	-0,536	1,69 g	Energy	0,180	2056 kcal
Mg	-0,484	310 mg	Cholesterol	0,110	279 mg
Ginger	-0,453	59 g			
Vitamin D	-0,446	6,26 mcg			
Omega-3 FA	-0,436	1,06 g			
Vitamin C	-0,424	118 mg			
Garlic	-0,412	4,35 g			

[*]Positive inflammation effective score = proinflammatory; negative inflammation effective score = antiinflammatory.

Table 1.
10 most effective antiinflammatory nutrients based on their activity level (inflammation effective score).

Authors/design of the study	Ethnicity/ participants	DII	Objectives	Main results
Shivappa N et al. 2014/prospective cohort	United States (Iowa)/34,703 postmenopausal women of the IWHS	DII based on 37 nutrient parameters	To examine association between DII (quintile) and CRC	Significantly higher risk for CRC in the 5th quintile (high DII)
Shivappa N et al. 2015/case-control study	Italy/326 patients with pancreatic carcinoma and 652 controls (median age 63 years)	DII based on 45 nutrient parameters	To analyze the association between the DII and the risk of pancreatic cancer	Subjects in the 2nd, 3rd, 4th and 5th quintiles had increased risk for pancreatic cancer
Mohseni R et al. 2018/ meta-analysis	Italy, Jamaica, France, Mexico, Iran, Canada/age span 40-94/*depending on publication	DII dependent on each publication/ DII is ranged between 18 and 36 nutrient parameters	To investigate relationship between DII and risk of developing prostate cancer	Men who had followed a pro-inflammatory diet were more at risk at developing prostate cancer
Zamora-Ros R et al. 2014/ case-control study	Spain/424 male participants and 401 control/age span 39-60	DII based on 37 nutrient parameters	To investigate association between DII and CRC and its interaction with polymorphisms of inflammatory genes	High DII diets are associated with increased risk of CRC association differed on the genotype of the cytokines
Tabung FK et al. 2014/prospective study	United States/161808 postmenopausal women	DII based on 45 nutrient parameters	To examine the association of DII with increased risk for CRC in WHI	Consumption of more DII diet was associated with increased risk of CRC, especially proximal colon
Schivappa N et al. 2016/case control study	Italy/454 women/age span 18-79	DII based on 45 nutrient parameters	To examine the association of DII with increased risk of endometrial cancer	Consumption of more DII diet was associated with increased risk of endometrial cancer
Schivappa N et al. 2015/case control study	Italy/258 participants/age span 43-84 years	DII based on 45 nutrient parameters	To examine the association of DII with increased risk for hepatocellular cancer	Consumption of more DII diet was associated with increased risk for hepatocellular cancer
Ghazizadeh H et al. 2020/cross sectional study	Iran/7083 adults of the MASHAD cohort study (age span 35-65 years)	DII based on 65 nutrient parameters	To quantify the possible inflammatory effect of diet on the occurrence of depression and anxiety	Significant association between 3rd and 4th quartiles of DII score with severe depression level

Authors/design of the study	Ethnicity/ participants	DII	Objectives	Main results
Salari-Moghaddam A et al. 2018/cross sectional study	Iran/3363 adult participants (age span 35-45 years)	DII based on 45 nutrient parameters	To examine the association between DII score and psychological disorders	Higher DII score was associated with anxiety and psychological distress
Ruiz-Canela M. et al. 2015/cross sectional study	Spain/7447 PREDIMED participants (men aged 55-80; women aged 60-80)	DII food parameter-specific for an individual	To examine the relationship between DII and indices of general and abdominal obesity	Pro-inflammatory diet is associated with central and abdominal obesity

DII and its correlation with carcinomas and other diseases.
IWHS - Iowa Women's Health Study; CRC – colorectal carcinoma; WHI - Women's Health Initiative; MASHAD -
Mashhad Stroke and Heart Atherosclerotic Disorder; PREDIMED - Prevención con Dieta Mediterránea.

Table 2.
Association between dietary inflammatory indeks with chronic diseases and cancers.

Authors/design of the study	Ethnicity/participants	DII	Objectives	Main results
Veronese N et al. 2017/longitudinal cohort study	North America/3648 participants (mean age 60.6 years)	DII based on 24 nutrient parameters	To investigate whether the DII scores are associated with increased risks of fractures	Higher DII scores are associated with higher incidence of fractures in women
Orchard T et al. 2016/ cross sectional study	United States/160191 postmenopausal women	DII based on 32 nutrient parameters	To examine DII in relation to risk of fracture and BMD	Lower risk of fractures in women with highest DII
Correa-Rodríguez M et al. 2018/cross sectional study	Spain/599 participants (age span 18-25)	DII based on 25 nutrient parameters	To investigate association between DII with bone health and obesity in young adults	DII is associated with obesity parameters but not to osteoporosis in adulthood
Shivappa N et al. 2015/ cross sectional study	Iran/160 postmenopausal women	DII based on 25 nutrient parameters	To examine the relationship between the DII and BMD in lumbar spine and femoral neck	No significant association between DII and femoral neck BMD

DII - Dietary Inflammatory Index; BMD - Bone Mineral Density.

Table 3.
Association between dietary inflammatory index (DII) with bone mineral density and fracture risk.

Proper nutrition based on the anti-inflammatory pyramid and changes in poor eating habits is a long-term strategy for preventing inflammation and developing osteoporosis. The level of inflammation can be measured and monitored using several biomarkers, including pro-and anti-inflammatory cytokines. The main pro-inflammatory cytokines are tumor necrosis factor (TNF), interleukin (IL) -1, L-6 and interferon (IFN). Anti-inflammatory cytokines are IL-4 and IL-10. C-reactive protein (CRP), and the more recently highly sensitive C-reactive protein (hs-CRP), are clinical markers of inflammation that were used in the study that investigated the association between different conditions and levels of inflammation [37].

Proinflammatory cytokines such as TNF-α, NF-κB, IL-1, and IL-6 are key mediators of the osteoclast differentiation and bone resorption. Bone resorption and bone loss due to chronic inflammation and increased proinflammatory cytokines is found in patients with periodontitis [38], pancreatitis [39] and rheumatoid arthritis [40]. It is also been established that upregulated proinflammatory cytokines are primary mediators of osteopenia or osteoporosis. These proinflammatory cytokines stimulate osteoclast activity through the regulation of the RANKL/RANK/OPG pathway [41]. The assorted increase within the event of osteoarthritis in obese human subjects is another evidence that chronic inflammation influences bone metabolism.

Since the introduction of the inflammatory diet index, numerous studies have related this method to bone health (**Table 3**). All the investigations represented in **Table 3** have analyzed relationship between DII and BMD or fracture risk and results are inconclusive. In a study of Rodrigez et al., association between DII and obesity in young adults was found, with no implication for bone health. Even though, there are rising evidences that in elderly women fat tissue can compromise bone structure and quality. Accordingly, some clinical data showed that obesity is not always protective against osteoporosis. This is supported by the fact that in obesity BMD values are usually falsely increased due to fat deposition and incorrect positioning during bone densitometry scanning [42, 43]. More adequate interpretation of the bone mass has been given by NMR imaging, which revealed decreased values of the trabecular bone volume in elderly women, due to bone marrow infiltration with fat. Given the fact that postmenopausal women have more bone marrow fat in the forearm bones, their trabecular bone volume is deteriorated, which could lead to bone fracture [42]. Replacement of the osteoblasts with adipocytes due to aging or hormones deprivation can also occur as a result of immobilization or physical inactivity. The results of the experimental studies suggest that obesity is epigenetic factor, which can compromise new bone formation in a male offspring of fat mothers. The possible mechanism that prevents bone formation includes systemic inflammation and activation of the RANK/RANKL/OPG system [21, 22]. Pro-inflammatory cytokines, such as TNF-α, activate NF-κB from fat cells in obesity, which could affect bone metabolism in a manner of enhanced bone resorption mediated by osteoclasts and sRANKL [21, 22].

3. Conclusion

Considering everything, it is clear that further clinical randomized studies are needed to better understand the influence of DII on bone mineral density. Of utmost importance are prospective studies that will follow up dietary habits (DII) along with concentrations of the bone remodeling markers as dynamic indicators of the bone metabolism.

Special attention should be given to obese patients who are at one hand prone to osteoporosis due to increased production of the proinflammatory cytokines from the fat tissue and, on the other hand, lower concentrations of the vitamin D in serum [38]. DII and bone remodeling markers should be followed in patients who lose and gain weight to better understand the influence of the inflammatory diet on bone metabolism and to answer the question, whether an anti-inflammatory diet has a positive impact on bone health.

Acknowledgements

The chapter was published from the funds of the Rijeka City Department of Health and Social Welfare and the Municipality of Kostrena Department of Health Welfare.

Conflict of interest

"The authors declare no conflict of interest."

Appendix and nomenclature

sRANKL	solubile receptor activator of nuclear factor κ-B ligand
RANK	receptor activator of nuclear factor κB
OPG	osteoprotegerin
WHO	World Health Organization
DEXA	dual- energy X-ray absorptiometry
BMD	bone mineral density
SD	standard deviations
TRAP	tartrate-resistant acid phosphatase
CTx	C-terminal telopeptide
NTx	N-terminal telopeptide
bALP	bone-specific alkaline phosphatase
TNF-α	tumor necrosis factor alpha
DII	Dietary Inflammatory Index
IL-6	interleukin 6
IL-4	interleukin 4
IL-10	interleukin 10
CRP	C-reactive protein
IFN	interferon
NFκB	nuclear factor-kappa B
NMR	nuclear magnetic resonance

Author details

Olga Cvijanović Peloza[1]*, Sandra Pavičić Žeželj[2], Gordana Kenđel Jovanović[2], Ivana Pavičić[3], Ana Terezija Jerbić Radetić[1], Sanja Zoričić Cvek[1], Jasna Lulić Drenjak[4], Gordana Starčević Klasan[1], Ariana Fužinac Smojver[5] and Juraj Arbanas[1]

1 Department of Anatomy, Medical Faculty of the University of Rijeka, Rijeka, Croatia

2 Department of Health Ecology, Medical Faculty of the University of Rijeka, Rijeka, Croatia

3 Clinic of Internal Medicine, CHC Rijeka, Rijeka, Croatia

4 Department of Physiotherapy, Faculty of Health Studies of the University of Rijeka, Rijeka, Croatia

5 Department of Basic Medical Sciences, Faculty of Health Studies of the University of Rijeka, Rijeka, Croatia

*Address all correspondence to: olga.cvijanovic@uniri.hr

IntechOpen

References

[1] Prentice A. Diet, nutrition and prevention of osteoporosis. Pub Health Nutr 2004; 7: 227-243.

[2] Department of Health and Human Services(HHS), Department of Agriculture(USDA). Dietary Guidelines for Americans, 2005.

[3] Antonić Degač K, Capak K, Kaić-Rak A, Kramarić D, Ljubičić M, Maver H, Mesaroš-Kanjski E, Petrović I., Reiner Ž. Hrvatska prehrambena politika. Ministarstvo zdravstva Republike Hrvatske, Hrvatski zavod za javno zdravstvo, 1999.

[4] Whitney E, Rolfes SR. Understanding Nutrition. Eleventh Edition. Belmont USA: Thomson. 2008, str.3,106.

[5] Šatalić Z. Povijest znanosti o prehrani. Medicus 2008;17(1):149-156.

[6] Mandić LM. Znanost o prehrani. Hrana i prehrana u čuvanju zdravlja. Osijek: Prehrambeno-tehnološki fakultet.2007, str.4, 57-91.

[7] Novotny R, Boushey C, Bock MA, Peck L, Auld G, Bruhn CM, Gustafson D, Gabel K, Jensen JK, Misner S, Read M. Calcium Intake of Asian, Hispanic and White Youth. J Am Coll Nutr 2003; 22:64-70.

[8] Pravilnik o hrani za posebne prehrambene potrebe 2004, Zagreb, Narodne novine, broj 81 (NN 81/04).

[9] Nieves JW. Osteoporosis: the role of micronutrients. Am J Clin Nutr 2005; 81: 1232S-1239S.

[10] Heaney RP. Nutrition and risk for osteoporosis. In: (Marcus R, Feldman D, Kelsey J, eds), Osteoporosis. San Diego: Academic Press, 1996:p.483-505.

[11] Rapuri PB, Gallagher JC, Haynatzka V. Protein intake: effects on bone mineral density and the rate of bone loss in elderly women. Am J Clin Nutr 2003;77:1517-1525.

[12] Gaffney-Stomberg E, Insogna KL, Rodriguez NR, Kerstetter JE. Increasing dietary protein requirements in elderly people for optimal muscle and bone health. J Am Geriatr Soc 2009;57(6):1073-1079.

[13] Zaidi, Mone & Buettner, Christoph & Sun, Li & Iqbal, Jameel. (2012). Minireview: The Link Between Fat and Bone: Does Mass Beget Mass?. Endocrinology. 153. 2070-2075. 10.1210/en.2012-1022.

[14] Magni P., Dozio E., Galliera E., Ruscica M., Corsi M. (2010) Molecular aspects of adipokine–bone interactions. Curr Mol Med 10: 522-532.

[15] Cao J. (2011) Effects of obesity on bone metabolism. J Orthop Surg Res 6: 30.

[16] Jessica K.Black, N.D. The Anti-Inflammation Diet and Recipe Book.

[17] Marshall D, Johnell O, Wedel H. Meta-analysis of how well measures of bone mineral density predict occurrence of osteoporotic fractures. BMJ 1996;312:1254-1259.

[18] Kanis JA, Borgstrom F, De Laet C i sur. A meta-analysis of previous fracture and subsequent fracture risk. Bone 2004;35:375-382.

[19] Xu J, Lombardi G, Jiao W, Banfi G. Effects of Exercise on Bone Status in Female Subjects, from Young Girls to Postmenopausal Women: An Overview of Systematic Reviews and Meta-Analyses. Sports Med. 2016;46(8):1165-1182. doi:10.1007/s40279-016-0494-0

[20] Watts NB. Clinical utility of biochemical markers of

bone remodeling. Clin Chem 1999;45:1359-1368.

[21] Mundy GR. Osteoporosis and inflammation. Nutr Rev. 2007;65(12 Pt 2):S147-S151. doi:10.1111/j.1753-4887.2007.tb00353.x

[22] Peric Kacarevic, Z., Snajder, D., Maric, A., Bijelic, N., Cvijanovic, O., Domitrovic, R., Radic, R. (2016). High-fat diet induced changes in lumbar vertebra of the male rat offsprings. Acta Histochemica, 118(7), 711-721. doi:10.1016/j.acthis.2016.08.002

[23] Shivappa N, Steck SE, Hurley TG i sur. Designing and developing a literature-derived, population-based dietary inflammatory index. Public Health Nutr. 2014;17(8):1689-1696;

[24] Shivappa N, Herbert JR, Rietzschel ER i sur. Associations between dietary inflammatory index and inflammatory markers in the Asklepios Study. Br J Nutr. 2015;113:665-671;

[25] Ruiz-Canela M, Bes-Rastrollo M, Martínez-González MA. The Role of Dietary Inflammatory Index in Cardiovascular Disease, Metabolic Syndrome and Mortality. Int. J. Mol. Sci. 2016;17(8):1265;

[26] Shivappa, N , Hébert JR, Zucchetto A i sur. Dietary inflammatory index and endometrial cancer risk in an Italian case-control study. Br J Nutr. 2016;115(1):138-146;

[27] Shivappa N, Hébert JR, Polesel J i sur. Inflammatory potential of diet and risk for hepatocellular cancer in a case-control study from Italy. Br J Nutr. 2016;115(2):324-331;

[28] Shivappa N, Prizment AE, Blair CK, Jacobs DR Jr, Steck SE, Hébert JR. Dietary inflammatory index and risk of colorectal cancer in the Iowa Women's Health Study. Cancer Epidemiol Biomarkers Prev. 2014

Nov;23(11):2383-92. doi: 10.1158/1055-9965.EPI-14-0537. Epub 2014 Aug 25. PMID: 25155761; PMCID: PMC4221503.

[29] Mohseni R, Abbasi S, Mohseni F, Rahimi F, Alizadeh S. Association between Dietary Inflammatory Index and the Risk of Prostate Cancer: A Meta-Analysis. Nutr Cancer. 2019;71(3):359-366. doi: 10.1080/01635581.2018.1516787. Epub 2018 Oct 1. PMID: 30273060.

[30] Shivappa N, Bosetti C, Zucchetto A, Serraino D, La Vecchia C, Hébert JR. Dietary inflammatory index and risk of pancreatic cancer in an Italian case-control study. Br J Nutr. 2015 Jan 28;113(2):292-8. doi: 10.1017/S0007114514003626. Epub 2014 Dec 17. PMID: 25515552; PMCID: PMC4470878.

[31] Zamora-Ros R, Shivappa N, Steck SE, Canzian F, Landi S, Alonso MH, Hébert JR, Moreno V. Dietary inflammatory index and inflammatory gene interactions in relation to colorectal cancer risk in the Bellvitge colorectal cancer case-control study. Genes Nutr. 2015 Jan;10(1):447. doi: 10.1007/s12263-014-0447-x. Epub 2014 Dec 9. PMID: 25488145; PMCID: PMC4259879.

[32] Tabung FK, Steck SE, Ma Y, Liese AD, Zhang J, Caan B, Hou L, Johnson KC, Mossavar-Rahmani Y, Shivappa N, Wactawski-Wende J, Ockene JK, Hebert JR. The association between dietary inflammatory index and risk of colorectal cancer among postmenopausal women: results from the Women's Health Initiative. Cancer Causes Control. 2015 Mar;26(3):399-408. doi: 10.1007/s10552-014-0515-y. Epub 2014 Dec 31. PMID: 25549833; PMCID: PMC4334706.

[33] Fowler ME, Akinyemiju TF. Meta-Analysis of the Association Between Dietary Inflammatory Index (DII) and Cancer Outcomes. Int J Cancer. 2017(prihvaćen manuskript. doi:10.1002/ijc.30922).

[34] Wood L, Shivappa N, Berthon BS i sur. Dietary inflammatory index is related to asthma risk, lung function and systemic inflammation in asthma. Clin Exp Allergy. 2015;45:177-183;

[35] Salari-Moghaddam A, Keshteli AH, Afshar H, Esmaillzadeh A, Adibi P. Association between dietary inflammatory index and psychological profile in adults. Clin Nutr. 2019 Oct;38(5):2360-2368. doi: 10.1016/j. clnu.2018.10.015. Epub 2018 Oct 27. PMID: 30415907.

[36] Ghazizadeh, H., Yaghooti-Khorasani, M., Asadi, Z. et al. Association between Dietary Inflammatory Index (DII®) and depression and anxiety in the Mashhad Stroke and Heart Atherosclerotic Disorder (MASHAD) Study population. BMC Psychiatry 20, 282 (2020). https://doi.org/10.1186/s12888-020-02663-4

[37] Nanri A, Moore MA, Kono S. Impact of C-reactive protein on disease risk and its relation to dietary factors. Asian Pac J Cancer Prev 2007;8:167-177.

[38] Van Dyke TE, Serhan CN. Resolution of inflammation: a new paradigm for the pathogenesis of periodontal diseases. J Dent Res. 2003 Feb;82(2):82-90. doi: 10.1177/154405910308200202. PMID: 12562878.

[39] Mann ST, Stracke H, Lange U, Klör HU, Teichmann J. Alterations of bone mineral density and bone metabolism in patients with various grades of chronic pancreatitis. Metabolism. 2003 May;52(5):579-585. doi: 10.1053/meta.2003.50112. PMID: 12759887.

[40] Romas E, Gillespie MT, Martin TJ. Involvement of receptor activator of NFκB ligand and tumor necrosis factor-α in bone destruction in rheumatoid arthritis, Bone, Volume 30, Issue 2, 2002, pages 340-346, ISSN 8756-3282.

[41] Khosla S. Minireview: the OPG/RANKL/RANK system. Endocrinology. 2001 Dec;142(12):5050-5055. doi: 10.1210/endo.142.12.8536. PMID: 11713196.

[42] Rosen CJ, Bouxsein ML. Mechanisms of disease: is osteoporosis the obesity of bone? Nat Clin Pract Rheumatol. 2006 Jan;2(1):35-43. doi: 10.1038/ncprheum0070. PMID: 16932650.

[43] Vanlint S. Vitamin D and Obesity. Nutrients. 2013; 5(3):949-956. https://doi.org/10.3390/nu5030949

Chapter 4

Osteoporosis: A Multifactorial Disease

Di Wu, Anna Cline-Smith, Elena Shashkova
and Rajeev Aurora

Abstract

A great achievement of modern medicine is the increased lifespan of the human population. Unfortunately, the comorbidities of aging have created a large economic and health burden on society. Osteoporosis is the most prevalent age-related disease. It is characterized by uncoupled bone resorption that leads to low bone mass, compromised microarchitecture and structural deterioration that increases the likelihood of fracture with minimal trauma, known as fragility fractures. These fractures lead to disproportionally high mortality rate and a drastic decline in quality of life for those affected. While estrogen loss is one known trigger of osteoporosis, a number of recent studies have shown that osteoporosis is a multifactorial condition in both humans and rodent models. The presence or absence of certain factors are likely to determine which subset of the population develop osteoporosis. In this chapter, we review the factors that contribute to osteoporosis with an emphasis on its multifactorial nature and the therapeutic consequences.

Keywords: osteoporosis, postmenopausal osteoporosis, aging, mineral homeostasis, gut microbiome, metabolism, osteoimmunology, therapy, T-cells

1. Introduction

Osteoporosis (OP) is the most prevalent metabolic bone disease that affects half the women and one third of men, typically, in the sixth and seventh decade of life [1, 2]. OP is characterized by uncoupled bone resorption that leads to low bone mass, compromised microarchitecture and structural deterioration that increases the likelihood of fractures with minimal trauma, known as fragility fractures. These fractures lead to disproportionally high mortality rate and a drastic decline in quality of life for those affected.

OP is diagnosed by an X-ray (typically by dual energy X-ray absorptiometry or DEXA) scan to measure bone mineral density (BMD) [3]. Two scores are returned: a Z-score and a T-score [4]. The T-score is normalized BMD by sex and age, whereas the Z-score also accounts for weight and ethnicity. Both scores report standard deviations (σ) of BMD from mean. A T-score of -1 is normal (within 1 σ of mean), whereas less than -1 to -2.5 indicates osteopenia. A patient with T-scores less than -2.5 is considered osteoporotic. Additional factors to BMD such as smoking, family history of fractures, the diagnosis of rheumatoid arthritis, alcohol consumption and glucocorticoid use many be considered to predict the probability of fracture using a fracture risk assessment tool score or FRAX score [5, 6].

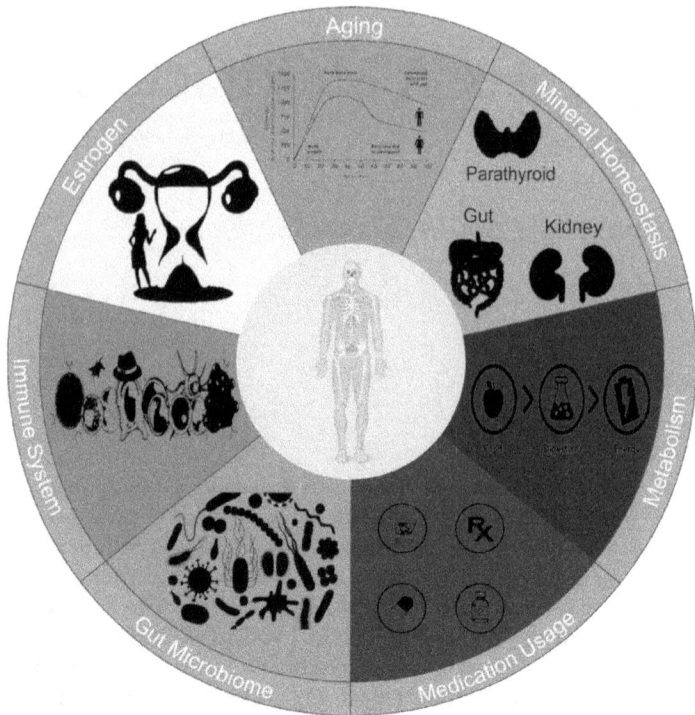

Figure 1.
The multifactorial nature of osteoporosis (OP). Osteoporosis is most commonly associated both aging and estrogen loss. This figure summarizes factors that affect bone health.

The skeletal system has several physiological functions. First, it provides mechanical support that allows for locomotion. Bone is weight bearing and serves as an anchor for muscle. Osteocytes are bone matrix embedded mechanosensory cells, that promote bone loss or gain (adaptation) to loads placed on the bone (i.e., Wolff's law). The marrow space within long bones serves as the primary site of hematopoiesis in an adult. When hematopoietic-derived cells are depleted in the periphery (due to inflammation, for instance) there is demand on the bone marrow [7, 8] to release both progenitors and differentiated cells into circulation [9, 10]. Bone also serves as the primary store for calcium and phosphate, and thus is under control of hormones produced by the parathyroid gland (parathyroid hormone or PTH and calcitonin) and kidneys (fibroblast growth factor 23 or FGF23). Vitamin D facilitate calcium absorption from the diet while PTH, calcitonin and FGF23 regulate serum calcium levels and responds to different physiological needs. In recent years, there is growing appreciation of the diverse roles the skeletal system plays in a person's health, including whole body metabolism, immune regulation and neurocognitive functions [11], in addition to the previously recognized roles of mechanical support and mineral homeostasis. Based on the function of the skeleton, OP can result from dysregulation in one or more factors that we will discuss in detail below (**Figure 1**).

2. Bone biology

Bone remodeling is a coordinated process where bone resorption and bone formation occur at the same location throughout life to repair microfractures and maintain bone homeostasis. Imbalances in bone remodeling underscore the pathophysiology of OP. There are three major cell types involved in bone remodeling: bone resorbing osteoclasts, bone forming osteoblasts, and osteocytes. Osteoclasts (OC) are multi-nucleated, bone-specialized macrophages, whose differentiation depends on receptor activator of nuclear factor kappa B (NF-κB) (RANK) and its ligand (RANKL). Osteoblasts (OB) differentiate from mesenchymal stem cells (MSC) and are responsible for bone formation. Many signaling pathways have been discovered that are critical for osteogenic differentiation, including Wingless and Int-1 (WNT)/β-catenin, bone morphogenic protein (BMP) and mechanistic target of rapamycin (mTOR). During bone remodeling, OC are recruited to the site of repair, where they will initiate bone resorption through two major mechanisms: 1) acidification of the microenvironment and 2) secretion of matrix metalloproteases. Towards the end of the resorption phase, OC will recruit MSC and osteoprogenitors and promote the differentiation and maturation of OB. At the same time, OB will secrete osteoprotegerin (OPG), a decoy receptor of RANKL, which will inhibit osteoclastogenesis and shut down bone resorption. OB will then begin producing extracellular matrix that will eventually calcify and become newly mineralized bone. As such, bone resorption and bone formation are tightly coupled and highly regulated. Together, OC and OB form the basic multicellular unit (BMU), the smallest functional unit during bone formation. During remodeling the OC and OB form the bone remodeling unit (BRU). Mature OB have three different fates when bone formation is complete. The majority will undergo apoptosis, a small fraction will become senescent bone lining cells, and an even smaller number become osteocytes. Osteocytes (Ocy) are stellate like cells embedded within mineralized bone that are mechanosensors within the bone. Ocy have a pivotal regulatory role in bone homeostasis, directing and coordinating fracture repair by regulating the BRU. Ocy they have recently been shown to have both osteolytic and anabolic functions and play a pivotal role during lactation [12].

3. Aging and osteoporosis

Both men and women develop OP [13]. The skeletal system grows rapidly post-natally and through puberty. Peak bone mass is attained by mid-third decade (mid 20s) of life [14]. Beginning at the end of the third decade, both sexes start to lose bone mass [14] that continues with aging. The rate (or slope = change in bone mass/change in time) varies by anatomical site [15] and by additional factors discussed in this chapter. It follows that the range between normal bone mass, osteopenia and OP is determined by both the peak bone mass (baseline) and the rate of age-related bone loss. Aging leads to increased senescent stem cells that repopulate OC and OB leading to deficiency in repair of microfractures that develop with use [16–18]. A recent study has shown that ablating senescent osteoclast precursors did not improve age-related bone loss [19]. There is accelerated bone loss (called the acute phase) in menopausal women [20–22]. The sex differences in age-related bone loss in humans can be recapitulated in mice [23]. In addition to the senescence of progenitor cells, increased oxidative stress during aging have been reported to decreased osteoblastogenesis while simultaneously increase osteoclastogenesis, favoring bone resorption [24]. Further research is needed to understand the effects of aging on bone and crosstalk with other factors.

4. Calcium, vitamin D3 and mineral homeostasis

It is standard practice to advise supplementation of calcium and vitamin D to osteoporotic women. However, most studies have shown that subjects of European ancestry are replete in calcium and vitamin D [25]. A number of studies and meta-analyses prior to 2010 showed an efficacy in reducing fracture risk with vitamin D alone, calcium alone and the combination [26, 27]. The lack of efficacy in some studies was attributed to lack of compliance [28]. There is a historical precedence that links rickets/osteomalacia and OP from the 17th century. The softening of bones became rampant in industrialized countries during the 19th century but rickets/osteomalacia were not clearly distinguished from OP until 1885. It was shown that rickets was due to the lack of new bone formation whereas OP was due to increased bone resorption [29]. Nonetheless, the overlap between hyperparathyroidism, under nourishment, calcium malabsorption with vitamin D insufficiency has become a paradigm for OP leading to practice of advising supplementation [30]. However, recent studies that have indicated that high serum calcium is associated with cardiovascular events, specifically stroke and increase coronary artery calcification, have led to questioning this practice [31–33]. This increase was due to supplementary calcium and not observed with natural dietary calcium [31, 32]. More recent meta-analysis found a trend for increased risk of cardiovascular events with calcium supplementation, although it was not statistically significant [34]. Additional studies are needed to resolve this question.

5. Body mass index (BMI) and metabolism

Epidemiological studies have shown elderly men and postmenopausal women with low BMI have lower T-scores and are classified as osteopenic or osteoporotic. A positive correlation has been observed in postmenopausal women between high BMI and prevalence of osteoarthritis (OA) and a negative correlation with prevalence of OP [35–37]. Adipocytes produce hormones (adipokines) that have been shown to regulate bone mass [38, 39]. Adipose tissue, especially visceral adipose tissue, has also been shown to harbor proinflammatory T-cells [40, 41]. Recently, Zou et al. showed that ablation of bone marrow adipocytes in mice cause a dramatic increase in bone mass [42]. Therefore, adipose tissue and obesity forms a complex link to bone health. First, white adipose tissue directly influences OB via adipokines [43]. Second, adipose tissue activates T-cells to produce proinflammatory cytokines tumor necrosis factor alpha (TNFα), interleukin (IL)-1β and IL-6. Additionally, insulin resistance is associated with obesity, thus altered glucose metabolism also affects bone metabolism, which has been shown to impede OB differentiation [44]. Further studies are needed to understand the mechanism(s) connecting inflammation, lipid and glucose metabolism to OA and OP.

6. Prescribed medicines contribute to osteoporosis

Recent studies have shown that patients taking certain commonly prescribed medicines have higher incidence of OP [45]. The best understood drug-induced bone loss is with glucocorticoids [46, 47]. There are also data suggesting that anticoagulants such as warfarin and heparin, which effect Vitamin K levels, are detrimental to bone health [48, 49]. This class of drugs also alters the gut microbiome adding to the complexity of interpretation [50]. Other drugs, including antiepileptics, proton pump inhibitors, opioid analgesics and aromatase inhibitors induce osteoporosis as well [51–54]. Further confounding the interpretation of data, these medications are often prescribed long-term in elderly populations who are already at risk due to age of osteoporosis. Even if the effect size of each medication is small, the combined drug–drug interactions can be more than additive [55, 56].

7. Modulation by the gut microbiome

The human digestive tract harbors trillions of microorganisms collectively known as the gut microbiome (GMB), which contain magnitudes more genetic information than our own genome. It is well recognized that the GMB plays an important role in educating the immune system, as germfree (GF) mice have reduced T cell populations. A number of studies have shown an association between GMB and bone health in both animal models [57, 58] and in humans [50]. However, Sjögrne et.al were the first to present evidence of direct interaction between the GMB and the bone [59]. They showed that GF mice had increased bone mass compared to conventionally raised (CONV-R) mice, and that transplantation of a GMB from CONV-R normalized bone mass. Since then, a number of studies have been conducted to investigate the regulation of bone homeostasis by the GMB. Estrogen (E_2) loss increases gut permeability [60–62], which leads to increased priming and activation of inflammation in the gut mucosa, leading to the generation of type 17 helper T-cells (Th17 cells). Segmented filamentous bacterium (SFB) have been shown to induce Th17 in the mice intestine and to promote decreased bone mass [63]. Th17 cells are potent inducers of osteoclastogenesis leading to increased bone resorption and bone loss. Li et al. demonstrated that bone loss in ovariectomized (OVX) mice is depended on the GMB and it can be prevented with supplementation of probiotics [64]. There is clear correlation between GMB and bone health, however the precise mechanisms remain elusive. Recent studies have suggested GMB produce microbial metabolites that have regulatory function on distal organs, including the bone. GMB derived butyrate, polyamines and short-chain fatty acids have been shown to induce regulatory T cell (T_{REG}) generation in the colon [65–67] and to regulate bone health. Thus, GMB modulate bone mass through a number of mechanisms, *viz.* by negatively by increasing Th17 cells, positively by inducing regulatory T-cells, and positively by producing metabolites that promote bone formation or inhibit bone resorption.

8. Chronic inflammation and regulation by the immune system

The recognition that T-cell derived cytokines affect bone has given rise to the field of osteoimmunology. The word *osteoimmunology* was first coined in 2000 by Arron and Choi [68], describing the crosstalk between the skeletal system and the immune system. Takayanagi et al. first reported such cross talk, demonstrating that T-cell produced interferon gamma (IFN-γ) can inhibit RANKL signaling during OC differentiation [69]. Since then, many studies have shown that TNFα and IL-17A promote osteoclastogenesis. Both cytokines are also increase in chronic inflammatory diseases such as rheumatoid arthritis, Crohn's, and some viral (i.e., human immunodeficiency virus or HIV) infections, which may explain why these patients have decreased bone mass [70–75]. TNFα has been shown to promote the production of RANKL from OB and osteocytes in addition to directly acting on OC precursors in synergy with RANKL [76–79]. PTH acts through T-cells to promote bone formation [80]. Th17 cells have been shown to increase osteoclastogenesis and resorption activity Th17 cells are the key pathogenic drive in immune-mediated bone destruction [81]. A number of studies have confirmed that IL-17A is a potent promoter of bone destruction, particularly in the context of autoimmune pathologies [82–84]. The field of osteoimmunology have thus far focused on OC, and additional studies are needed to assess how Th17 cells and the cytokines TNFα and IL-17A affect OB to limit bone formation. Inflammation has two effects: first, a direct effect where cytokines produced by T-cells act on the BRU to modulate bone homeostasis. Second, inflammation has an indirect effect that is due to increased demand on hematopoiesis. For instance, neutrophils and mast cells have short half-lives when they participate in inflammatory response. As they die, the immune cells are replenished by increased hematopoiesis and efflux of precursors and mature cells from the bone is mediated via regulation of osteoclastic activity [85–87]. The prolonged demand may also lead to bone erosion.

9. Postmenopausal osteoporosis

In women, aging leads to menopause, the cessation of ovarian function that is one of the leading causes of secondary osteoporosis. Early studies suggested that E_2 directly regulates OC [88–91] and OB [92, 93] and its loss at menopause results in long lived OC and impaired OB, and to uncoupled bone resorption [94]. Postmenopausal osteoporosis (PMOP) has been traditionally regarded as an endocrinal, E_2 deficiency mediated disease. Over the last two decades, it has become apparent that E_2-loss promotes persistent activation of T-cell that promotes acute phase of osteoporosis [80, 95, 96]. The mechanistic studies for linking E_2 loss at menopause and activation of the T-cells has come from ovariectomy (OVX) of rodents and key outcomes have been validated in human studies. OVX of female rodents is a well-established and widely used model for menopause. E_2 loss leads to both increased bone resorption and formation, however, this process is uncoupled where the former greatly exceeds the latter, resulting in net bone loss. Pacifici and colleagues first reported in 1990 that there is increased monocytic production of IL-1 in osteoporotic patients, indicating that in the absence of sex steroids, cytokines promote bone loss [97]. OVX of sexually mature mice that were T-cell

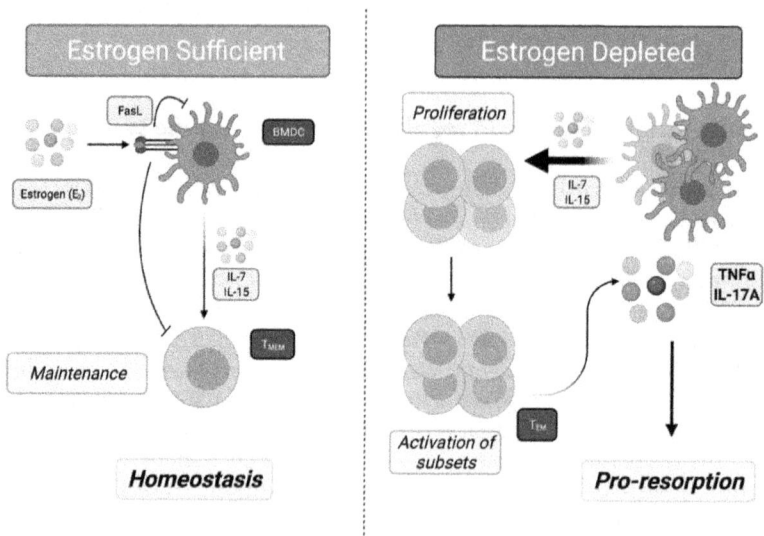

Figure 2.
Novel pathway of E_2 loss induced chronic inflammations leading to bone loss. Left panel: BMDC secrete IL-7, IL-15 or both to promote survival of T_{MEM}. E_2 induces FasL in the BMDC, resulting in shorter lifespans. In addition, IL-15 induces Fas in proliferating T_{MEM} in response to IL-7 and IL-15 thus maintain a homeostatic pool of T_{MEM}. Right panel: In absence of E_2, BMDC have reduced FasL expression, resulting in their proliferation and high concentrations of IL-7 and IL-15. Under these conditions, all T_{MEM} proliferate and a subset (~5 to 10%) become reactivated T_{EM} which produce TNFα and IL-17A, promoting bone resorption and also limits bone formation. BMDC = bone marrow resident dendritic cells, T_{MEM} = memory T-cells, T_{EM} = effector memory T-cells. This figure was created in BioRender.com

deficient showed decreased bone loss, which provided further evidence that T-cells play a key role in promoting bone resorption [98–102], as did blockade of TNFα [103] and IL-17A [104]. At the same time, Takayanagi et al. showed that IFN-γ regulated osteoclastogenesis [69, 105]. In the past decade, there is mounting evidence suggesting that the immune system and inflammation play a critical pathogenic role in uncoupled bone loss [82, 106–110].

Recently, our lab has described a new pathway where E_2 loss leads to chronic low-grade production of the proinflammatory cytokines TNFα and IL-17 by memory T-cells (T_{MEM}) that was dependent on IL-7 and IL-15 in mice [111] (**Figure 2**). The increased production of IL-7 and IL-15 was mediated by bone marrow dendritic cells (BMDCs), which in the absence of E_2 do not express FasL, leading to an antigen-independent activation of T_{MEM}. These T_{MEM} proliferate, and a subset become effector memory T-cells (T_{EM}) to produce TNFα and IL-17A. T_{MEM} encode a lifetime of exposures to antigens and only a subset of these could be converted to IL-17A and TNFα expressing. This notion would explain the variance at the population level in the development of PMOP. We hypothesize that the difference in the bone marrow T_{MEM} population based on the life-time antigen exposure would result in varying sensitivity of reactivation.

10. Therapeutics

The therapeutics prescribed most commonly for osteoporosis are anti-resorptives like bisphosphonates or denosumab. One issue with this class of medications are the adverse effects, most notably osteonecrosis of the jaw (ONJ). Although ONJ is rare (1–3%), it has been observed with anti-resorptive therapies (both bisphosphonates and denosumab) in patients with certain predisposing factors (i.e., after tooth extraction or in people with type 2 diabetes).

The second class of therapies are bone anabolics. Two examples of this class are teriparatide [112] and more recently romosozumab that targets sclerostin [113]. The bone anabolic therapies are also limited in their use because of potential adverse effects with prolonged use [114–116] and in special populations as well [117]. Furthermore, there is a limited window for the efficacy of many bone anabolic therapies due to adaptations in the bone in response to therapy. Interestingly, it has been observed in randomized control trials that the sequence of medication has substantial impacts on the long-term outcome. Patients who received teriparatide for 2 years first, followed by anti-resorptives maintained bone mass significantly longer than patient who received antiresorptives first [118].

As we discussed in this chapter, OP can arise from a combination of multiple causes. It follows that the treatment of osteoporosis should target additional mechanisms. All current therapies target the cells of the BRU, to suppress resorption of to promote bone formation. Furthermore, the current therapies have shortcomings and adverse effects with prolonged use necessitating drug holidays [119]. Therefore, additional therapies are needed, including a more precision medicine approach to treat osteoporosis. Immunomodulatory options such as anti-TNFα, anti-IL-17A and anti-RANKL have yielded inconsistent results in patients. Recently, Chong et al. [120] showed that neutralization of IL-17A induces compensatory increase of other Th17 cytokines, including IL-17F, IL-22 and GM-CSF. This has implication for the use of immunomodulatory therapies in PMOP.

Our laboratory discovered that OC are antigen presenting cells that induce Forkhead box protein 3 (FoxP3), cluster of differentiation (CD) 25, cytotoxic T-lymphocyte-associated protein (CTLA) 4 and expression of IFN-γ and IL-10 in $CD8^+$ T-cells in vitro (**Figure 3**). We have validated that these $CD8^+$ regulatory

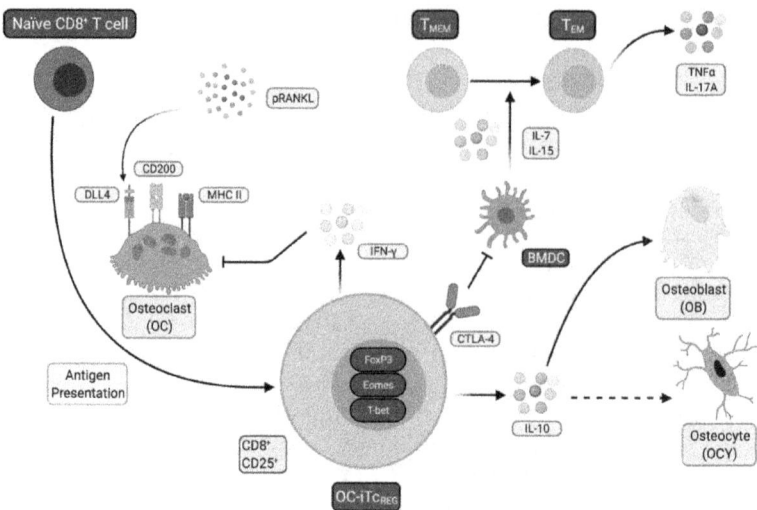

Figure 3.
Osteoclasts induce tolerogenic Tc_{REG}. OC use three signals to induce Tc_{REG}: Antigen-loaded MHC I, CD200 (a costimulation molecule that activates NF-κB) and the notch ligand DLL4. Treatment with pRANKL leads to increased expression DLL4 and therefore increased induction of Tc_{REG}. Tc_{REG} secrete IFN-γ that suppress osteoclastogenesis by degrading TRAF6 and resorption by mature OC. Tc_{REG} also secrete IL-10, which is required for the bone anabolic activity but not resolution of inflammation. IL-10 may also target Ocy to improve cortical bone mass. Resolution of inflammation appears to be mediated by CTLA4 expressed on Tc_{REG}. This figure was created in BioRender.com.

T-cell (Tc_{REG}) are induced by OC during bone resorption in vivo [121, 122]. Bone resorbing OC induce Tc_{REG} and Tc_{REG} suppress bone resorption by OC to form a negative feedback loop [123]. Tc_{REG} are also immunosuppressive like their CD4+ counter parts [124]. Both in vivo induction by low dose pulse RANKL (pRANKL) and adoptive transfer of ex vivo generated Tc_{REG} suppressed bone resorption, TNFα production and promoted bone formation to ameliorate osteoporosis in OVX mice [125]. In unpublished studies, OVX IL-10 deficient mice were unresponsive to the bone anabolic effects of pRANKL. However, Tc_{REG} retained its ability to inhibit TNFα production in T_{EM}, suggesting that the immunosuppressive effects are IL-10 independent. Further investigation showed that IL-10 directly regulates OB at the gene expression level. Taken together, our observations indicate that the immune system plays a fundamental role in modulating bone homeostasis, able to tip the balance either in favor of uncoupled bone resorption or bone formation.

11. Conclusions

In this chapter, we highlighted the multifactorial nature of osteoporosis. Bone loss occurs with age and slope associated with this decline may be enhanced with decreased vitamin D3, calcium deficiency in diet, medicines and polypharmacy, excess secretion of phosphate by kidneys, by hyperparathyroidism, chronic inflammation by persistent infections and autoimmune disease. E_2 loss also triggers a low-grade persistent inflammation in a subset of memory T-cells that promotes rapid bone erosion. Emerging evidence demonstrates significant interplay between these factors revealing the tradeoffs between organismal homeostasis and organ-specific regulation. Research in current decade is likely to provide new insights and mechanisms into the crosstalk. Revealing the mechanistic details will provide

Osteoporosis: A Multifactorial Disease
DOI: http://dx.doi.org/10.5772/intechopen.97549

exciting new targets for therapies. Furthermore, determining the factors in each individual would allow for precision medicine approach to promoting bone health in the aging population.

Acknowledgements

We thank Daniel Goering, Yiyi Zhang and Lizzie Geerling for contributing to additional unpublished experiments referenced herein.

Author Contributions

RA conceived of the manuscript. DW and RA drafted the manuscript. ACS and ES provided literature search and edits. All authors were involved in scientific discussion of the review.

Conflict of interest

The authors declare no conflict of interest.

Appendices

Appendix 1: Abbreviations

DEXA	dual energy X-ray absorptiometry
BMD	bone mineral density
FRAX	fracture risk assessment tool
PTH	parathyroid hormone
FGF23	fibroblast growth factor 23
OC	osteoclasts
NF-κB	nuclear factor kappa B
RANK	receptor activator of NF-κB
RANKL	receptor activator of NF-κB ligand
OB	osteoblasts
MSC	mesenchymal stem cells
WNT	wingless and Int-1
BMP	bone morphogenic protein
mTOR	mechanistic target of rapamycin
OPG	osteoprotegerin
BMU	basic multicellular unit
BRU	bone remodeling unit
BIM	body mass index
OA	osteoarthritis
TNFα	tumor necrosis factor alpha
IL	interleukin
GMB	gut microbiome
CONV-R	conventionally raised
Th	helper T cell
OVX	ovariectomy (surgery) or ovariectomized

T_{REG}	regulatory T cell
IFNγ	interferon gamma
HIV	human immunodeficiency virus
T_{MEM}	memory T cell
BMDC	bone marrow dendritic cells
T_{EM}	effector memory T cell
ONJ	osteonecrosis of the jaw
FoxP3	forkhead box P3
CD	cluster of differentiation
CTLA4	cytotoxic T-lymphocyte-associated protein 4

Author details

Di Wu, Anna Cline-Smith, Elena Shashkova and Rajeev Aurora*
Department of Molecular Microbiology and Immunology, Saint Louis University
School of Medicine, St. Louis, MO, USA

*Address all correspondence to: rajeev.aurora@health.slu.edu

IntechOpen

References

[1] Melton LJ. The prevalence of osteoporosis: gender and racial comparison. Calcified tissue international. 2001;69(4):179.

[2] Wright NC, Looker AC, Saag KG, Curtis JR, Delzell ES, Randall S, et al. The recent prevalence of osteoporosis and low bone mass in the United States based on bone mineral density at the femoral neck or lumbar spine. Journal of Bone and Mineral Research. 2014;29(11):2520-2526.

[3] Authority VIAE. Dual energy x-ray absorptiometry for bone mineral density and body composition assessment. 2010.

[4] Sahota O, Pearson D, Cawte SW, San P, Hosking DJ. Site-Specific Variation in the Classification of Osteoporosis, and the Diagnostic Reclassification Using the Lowest Individual Lumbar Vertebra T-score Compared with the L1–L4 Mean, in Early Postmenopausal Women. Osteoporosis International. 2000;11(10):852-857.

[5] Kanis JA, Borgstrom F, De Laet C, Johansson H, Johnell O, Jonsson B, et al. Assessment of fracture risk. Osteoporos Int. 2005;16(6):581-589.

[6] Kanis JA, Johnell O, Oden A, De Laet C, de Terlizzi F. Ten-year probabilities of clinical vertebral fractures according to phalangeal quantitative ultrasonography. Osteoporos Int. 2005;16(9): 1065-1070.

[7] Kuznetsov SA, Riminucci M, Ziran N, Tsutsui TW, Corsi A, Calvi L, et al. The interplay of osteogenesis and hematopoiesis: expression of a constitutively active PTH/PTHrP receptor in osteogenic cells perturbs the establishment of hematopoiesis in bone and of skeletal stem cells in the bone

marrow. J Cell Biol. 2004;167(6): 1113-1122.

[8] Yahata T, Muguruma Y, Yumino S, Sheng Y, Uno T, Matsuzawa H, et al. Quiescent human hematopoietic stem cells in the bone marrow niches organize the hierarchical structure of hematopoiesis. Stem Cells. 2008;26(12):3228-3236.

[9] Wilson A, Trumpp A. Bone-marrow haematopoietic-stem-cell niches. Nat Rev Immunol. 2006;6(2):93-106.

[10] Heideveld E, van den Akker E. Digesting the role of bone marrow macrophages on hematopoiesis. Immunobiology. 2017;222(6):814-822.

[11] Karsenty G, Ferron M. The contribution of bone to whole-organism physiology. Nature. 2012; 481(7381):314-320.

[12] Tsourdi E, Jähn K, Rauner M, Busse B, Bonewald LF. Physiological and pathological osteocytic osteolysis. Journal of musculoskeletal & neuronal interactions. 2018;18(3):292-303.

[13] Bonnick SL. Osteoporosis in men and women. Clin Cornerstone. 2006;8(1):28-39.

[14] Burr DB. Muscle strength, bone mass, and age-related bone loss. Journal of bone and mineral research. 1997;12(10):1547-1551.

[15] Aerssens J, Boonen S, Joly J, Dequeker J. Variations in trabecular bone composition with anatomical site and age: potential implications for bone quality assessment. J Endocrinol. 1997;155(3):411-421.

[16] Lopez-Otin C, Blasco MA, Partridge L, Serrano M, Kroemer G. The hallmarks of aging. Cell. 2013;153(6):1194-1217.

[17] Laurent MR, Dedeyne L, Dupont J, Mellaerts B, Dejaeger M, Gielen E. Age-related bone loss and sarcopenia in men. Maturitas. 2019;122:51-56.

[18] Morgan EF, Unnikrisnan GU, Hussein AI. Bone Mechanical Properties in Healthy and Diseased States. Annu Rev Biomed Eng. 2018;20:119-143.

[19] Kim HN, Chang J, Iyer S, Han L, Campisi J, Manolagas SC, et al. Elimination of senescent osteoclast progenitors has no effect on the age-associated loss of bone mass in mice. Aging Cell. 2019;18(3):e12923.

[20] Riggs BL. The mechanisms of estrogen regulation of bone resorption. J Clin Invest. 2000;106(10):1203-1204.

[21] Riggs BL, Khosla S, Atkinson EJ, Dunstan CR, Melton LJ, 3rd. Evidence that type I osteoporosis results from enhanced responsiveness of bone to estrogen deficiency. Osteoporos Int. 2003;14(9):728-733.

[22] Riggs BL, Khosla S, Melton LJ, 3rd. A unitary model for involutional osteoporosis: estrogen deficiency causes both type I and type II osteoporosis in postmenopausal women and contributes to bone loss in aging men. J Bone Miner Res. 1998;13(5):763-773.

[23] Glatt V, Canalis E, Stadmeyer L, Bouxsein ML. Age-related changes in trabecular architecture differ in female and male C57BL/6J mice. J Bone Miner Res. 2007;22(8):1197-1207.

[24] Ucer S, Iyer S, Kim HN, Han L, Rutlen C, Allison K, et al. The Effects of Aging and Sex Steroid Deficiency on the Murine Skeleton Are Independent and Mechanistically Distinct. J Bone Miner Res. 2017;32(3):560-574.

[25] Ringe JD. Plain vitamin D or active vitamin D in the treatment of osteoporosis: where do we stand today? Arch Osteoporos. 2020;15(1):182.

[26] Nordin BE. Evolution of the calcium paradigm: the relation between vitamin D, serum calcium and calcium absorption. Nutrients. 2010;2(9): 997-1004.

[27] Nowson CA. Prevention of fractures in older people with calcium and vitamin D. Nutrients. 2010;2(9):975-984.

[28] Hill TR, Aspray TJ, Francis RM. Vitamin D and bone health outcomes in older age. Proc Nutr Soc. 2013;72(4): 372-380.

[29] Pommer DG. Untersuchungen über Osteomalacie und Rachitis nebst Beiträgen zur Kenntniss der Knochenresorption und-apposition in verschiedenen Altersperioden und der durchbohrenden Gefässe, von Dr Gustav Pommer: FCW Vogel; 1885.

[30] Need AG, O'Loughlin PD, Morris HA, Coates PS, Horowitz M, Nordin BE. Vitamin D metabolites and calcium absorption in severe vitamin D deficiency. J Bone Miner Res. 2008;23(11):1859-1863.

[31] Anderson JJ, Kruszka B, Delaney JA, He K, Burke GL, Alonso A, et al. Calcium Intake From Diet and Supplements and the Risk of Coronary Artery Calcification and its Progression Among Older Adults: 10-Year Follow-up of the Multi-Ethnic Study of Atherosclerosis (MESA). J Am Heart Assoc. 2016;5(10).

[32] Li K, Kaaks R, Linseisen J, Rohrmann S. Associations of dietary calcium intake and calcium supplementation with myocardial infarction and stroke risk and overall cardiovascular mortality in the Heidelberg cohort of the European Prospective Investigation into Cancer and Nutrition study (EPIC-Heidelberg). Heart. 2012;98(12):920-925.

[33] Hulbert M, Turner ME, Hopman WM, Anastassiades T,

Adams MA, Holden RM. Changes in vascular calcification and bone mineral density in calcium supplement users from the Canadian Multi-center Osteoporosis Study (CaMOS). Atherosclerosis. 2020;296:83-90.

[34] Jenkins DJA, Spence JD, Giovannucci EL, Kim YI, Josse R, Vieth R, et al. Supplemental Vitamins and Minerals for CVD Prevention and Treatment. J Am Coll Cardiol. 2018;71(22):2570-2584.

[35] Chen Z, Klimentidis YC, Bea JW, Ernst KC, Hu C, Jackson R, et al. Body Mass Index, Waist Circumference, and Mortality in a Large Multiethnic Postmenopausal Cohort-Results from the Women's Health Initiative. J Am Geriatr Soc. 2017;65(9):1907-1915.

[36] Ichchou L, Allali F, Rostom S, Bennani L, Hmamouchi I, Abourazzak FZ, et al. Relationship between spine osteoarthritis, bone mineral density and bone turn over markers in post menopausal women. BMC Womens Health. 2010;10:25.

[37] Wright NC, Riggs GK, Lisse JR, Chen Z, Women's Health I. Self-reported osteoarthritis, ethnicity, body mass index, and other associated risk factors in postmenopausal women-results from the Women's Health Initiative. J Am Geriatr Soc. 2008;56(9): 1736-1743.

[38] Liu Z, Liu H, Li Y, Wang Y, Xing R, Mi F, et al. Adiponectin inhibits the differentiation and maturation of osteoclasts via the mTOR pathway in multiple myeloma. Int J Mol Med. 2020;45(4):1112-1120.

[39] Yang J, Park OJ, Kim J, Han S, Yang Y, Yun CH, et al. Adiponectin Deficiency Triggers Bone Loss by Up-Regulation of Osteoclastogenesis and Down-Regulation of Osteoblastogenesis. Front Endocrinol (Lausanne). 2019;10:815.

[40] Kintscher U, Hartge M, Hess K, Foryst-Ludwig A, Clemenz M, Wabitsch M, et al. T-lymphocyte infiltration in visceral adipose tissue: a primary event in adipose tissue inflammation and the development of obesity-mediated insulin resistance. Arteriosclerosis, thrombosis, and vascular biology. 2008;28(7): 1304-1310.

[41] Maury E, Brichard S. Adipokine dysregulation, adipose tissue inflammation and metabolic syndrome. Molecular and cellular endocrinology. 2010;314(1):1-16.

[42] Zou W, Rohatgi N, Brestoff JR, Li Y, Barve RA, Tycksen E, et al. Ablation of Fat Cells in Adult Mice Induces Massive Bone Gain. Cell Metab. 2020;32(5):801-13.e6.

[43] de Paula FJA, Rosen CJ. Marrow Adipocytes: Origin, Structure, and Function. Annu Rev Physiol. 2020;82: 461-484.

[44] Wei J, Shimazu J, Makinistoglu MP, Maurizi A, Kajimura D, Zong H, et al. Glucose Uptake and Runx2 Synergize to Orchestrate Osteoblast Differentiation and Bone Formation. Cell. 2015;161(7):1576-1591.

[45] Nguyen KD, Bagheri B, Bagheri H. Drug-induced bone loss: a major safety concern in Europe. Expert Opin Drug Saf. 2018;17(10):1005-1014.

[46] Kline GA, Morin SN, Lix LM, Leslie WD. Bone densitometry categories as a salient distracting feature in the modern clinical pathways of osteoporosis care: A retrospective 20-year cohort study. Bone. 2021;145:115861.

[47] Sandru F, Carsote M, Dumitrascu MC, Albu SE, Valea A. Glucocorticoids and Trabecular Bone Score. J Med Life. 2020;13(4): 449-453.

[48] Signorelli SS, Scuto S, Marino E, Giusti M, Xourafa A, Gaudio A. Anticoagulants and Osteoporosis. Int J Mol Sci. 2019;20(21).

[49] Dadwal G, Schulte-Huxel T, Kolb G. Effect of antithrombotic drugs on bone health. Z Gerontol Geriatr. 2020;53(5): 457-462.

[50] Das M, Cronin O, Keohane DM, Cormac EM, Nugent H, Nugent M, et al. Gut microbiota alterations associated with reduced bone mineral density in older adults. Rheumatology (Oxford). 2019;58(12):2295-2304.

[51] Ghebre YT. Proton Pump Inhibitors and Osteoporosis: Is Collagen a Direct Target? Front Endocrinol (Lausanne). 2020;11:473.

[52] Huang YL, Tsay WI, Her SH, Ho CH, Tsai KT, Hsu CC, et al. Chronic pain and use of analgesics in the elderly: a nationwide population-based study. Arch Med Sci. 2020;16(3): 627-634.

[53] Byreddy DV, Bouchonville MF, 2nd, Lewiecki EM. Drug-induced osteoporosis: from Fuller Albright to aromatase inhibitors. Climacteric. 2015;18 Suppl 2:39-46.

[54] Miller AS, Ferastraoaru V, Tabatabaie V, Gitlevich TR, Spiegel R, Haut SR. Are we responding effectively to bone mineral density loss and fracture risks in people with epilepsy? Epilepsia Open. 2020;5(2):240-247.

[55] Al-Qurain AA, Gebremichael LG, Khan MS, Williams DB, Mackenzie L, Phillips C, et al. Prevalence and Factors Associated with Analgesic Prescribing in Poly-Medicated Elderly Patients. Drugs Aging. 2020;37(4):291-300.

[56] Oshiro CES, Frankland TB, Rosales AG, Perrin NA, Bell CL, Lo SHY, et al. Fall Ascertainment and Development of a Risk Prediction Model

Using Electronic Medical Records. J Am Geriatr Soc. 2019;67(7):1417-1422.

[57] Ohlsson C, Engdahl C, Fåk F, Andersson A, Windahl SH, Farman HH, et al. Probiotics protect mice from ovariectomy-induced cortical bone loss. PLoS One. 2014;9(3):e92368.

[58] Britton RA, Irwin R, Quach D, Schaefer L, Zhang J, Lee T, et al. Probiotic L. reuteri treatment prevents bone loss in a menopausal ovariectomized mouse model. J Cell Physiol. 2014;229(11):1822-1830.

[59] Sjögren K, Engdahl C, Henning P, Lerner UH, Tremaroli V, Lagerquist MK, et al. The gut microbiota regulates bone mass in mice. J Bone Miner Res. 2012;27(6):1357-1367.

[60] Sabui S, Skupsky J, Kapadia R, Cogburn K, Lambrecht NW, Agrawal A, et al. Tamoxifen-induced, intestinal-specific deletion of Slc5a6 in adult mice leads to spontaneous inflammation: involvement of NF-kappaB, NLRP3, and gut microbiota. Am J Physiol Gastrointest Liver Physiol. 2019;317(4):G518-GG30.

[61] Roomruangwong C, Carvalho AF, Geffard M, Maes M. The menstrual cycle may not be limited to the endometrium but also may impact gut permeability. Acta Neuropsychiatr. 2019;31(6):294-304.

[62] Rizzetto L, Fava F, Tuohy KM, Selmi C. Connecting the immune system, systemic chronic inflammation and the gut microbiome: The role of sex. J Autoimmun. 2018;92:12-34.

[63] Ivanov II, Atarashi K, Manel N, Brodie EL, Shima T, Karaoz U, et al. Induction of Intestinal Th17 Cells by Segmented Filamentous Bacteria. Cell. 2009;139(3):485-498.

[64] Li JY, Chassaing B, Tyagi AM, Vaccaro C, Luo T, Adams J, et al.

Sex steroid deficiency-associated bone loss is microbiota dependent and prevented by probiotics. J Clin Invest. 2016;126(6):2049-2063.

[65] Furusawa Y, Obata Y, Fukuda S, Endo TA, Nakato G, Takahashi D, et al. Commensal microbe-derived butyrate induces the differentiation of colonic regulatory T cells. Nature. 2013;504(7480):446-450.

[66] Smith PM, Howitt MR, Panikov N, Michaud M, Gallini CA, Bohlooly YM, et al. The microbial metabolites, short-chain fatty acids, regulate colonic Treg cell homeostasis. Science. 2013;341(6145):569-573.

[67] Chevalier C, Kieser S, Colakoglu M, Hadadi N, Brun J, Rigo D, et al. Warmth Prevents Bone Loss Through the Gut Microbiota. Cell Metab. 2020;32(4): 575-90e7.

[68] Arron JR, Choi Y. Bone versus immune system. Nature. 2000;408 (6812):535-536.

[69] Takayanagi H, Ogasawara K, Hida S, Chiba T, Murata S, Sato K, et al. T-cell-mediated regulation of osteoclastogenesis by signalling cross-talk between RANKL and IFN-gamma. Nature. 2000;408 (6812):600-605.

[70] Blaschke M, Koepp R, Cortis J, Komrakova M, Schieker M, Hempel U, et al. IL-6, IL-1beta, and TNF-alpha only in combination influence the osteoporotic phenotype in Crohn's patients via bone formation and bone resorption. Adv Clin Exp Med. 2018;27(1):45-56.

[71] Sapir-Koren R, Livshits G. Postmenopausal osteoporosis in rheumatoid arthritis: The estrogen deficiency-immune mechanisms link. Bone. 2017;103:102-115.

[72] Klingberg E, Geijer M, Gothlin J, Mellstrom D, Lorentzon M, Hilme E,

et al. Vertebral fractures in ankylosing spondylitis are associated with lower bone mineral density in both central and peripheral skeleton. J Rheumatol. 2012;39(10):1987-1995.

[73] Shaiykova A, Pasquet A, Goujard C, Lion G, Durand E, Bayan T, et al. Reduced bone mineral density among HIV-infected, virologically controlled young men: prevalence and associated factors. AIDS. 2018;32(18):2689-2696.

[74] Moran CA, Weitzmann MN, Ofotokun I. Bone Loss in HIV Infection. Curr Treat Options Infect Dis. 2017;9(1):52-67.

[75] Piodi LP, Poloni A, Ulivieri FM. Managing osteoporosis in ulcerative colitis: something new? World J Gastroenterol. 2014;20(39):14087-14098.

[76] Zhao B, Grimes SN, Li S, Hu X, Ivashkiv LB. TNF-induced osteoclastogenesis and inflammatory bone resorption are inhibited by transcription factor RBP-J. The Journal of experimental medicine. 2012;209(2):319-334.

[77] Azuma Y, Kaji K, Katogi R, Takeshita S, Kudo A. Tumor Necrosis Factor-α Induces Differentiation of and Bone Resorption by Osteoclasts. Journal of Biological Chemistry. 2000;275(7):4858-4864.

[78] Kobayashi K, Takahashi N, Jimi E, Udagawa N, Takami M, Kotake S, et al. Tumor Necrosis Factor α Stimulates Osteoclast Differentiation by a Mechanism Independent of the Odf/Rankl–Rank Interaction. Journal of Experimental Medicine. 2000;191(2):275-286.

[79] Lam J, Takeshita S, Barker JE, Kanagawa O, Ross FP, Teitelbaum SL. TNF-α induces osteoclastogenesis by direct stimulation of macrophages exposed to permissive levels of RANK

ligand. The Journal of Clinical Investigation. 2000;106(12):1481-1488.

[80] Yu M, D'Amelio P, Tyagi AM, Vaccaro C, Li JY, Hsu E, et al. Regulatory T cells are expanded by Teriparatide treatment in humans and mediate intermittent PTH-induced bone anabolism in mice. EMBO Rep. 2018;19(1):156-171.

[81] Sato K, Suematsu A, Okamoto K, Yamaguchi A, Morishita Y, Kadono Y, et al. Th17 functions as an osteoclastogenic helper T cell subset that links T cell activation and bone destruction. J Exp Med. 2006;203(12): 2673-2682.

[82] Tyagi AM, Srivastava K, Mansoori MN, Trivedi R, Chattopadhyay N, Singh D. Estrogen deficiency induces the differentiation of IL-17 secreting Th17 cells: a new candidate in the pathogenesis of osteoporosis. PLoS One. 2012;7(9):e44552.

[83] Komatsu N, Okamoto K, Sawa S, Nakashima T, Oh-hora M, Kodama T, et al. Pathogenic conversion of Foxp3+ T cells into TH17 cells in autoimmune arthritis. Nat Med. 2014;20(1):62-68.

[84] Zhao R, Wang X, Feng F. Upregulated Cellular Expression of IL-17 by CD4+ T-Cells in Osteoporotic Postmenopausal Women. Annals of nutrition & metabolism. 2016;68(2): 113-118.

[85] Kollet O, Dar A, Lapidot T. The multiple roles of osteoclasts in host defense: bone remodeling and hematopoietic stem cell mobilization. Annu Rev Immunol. 2007;25:51-69.

[86] Kollet O, Dar A, Shivtiel S, Kalinkovich A, Lapid K, Sztainberg Y, et al. Osteoclasts degrade endosteal components and promote mobilization of hematopoietic progenitor cells. Nat Med. 2006;12(6):657-664.

[87] Mansour A, Abou-Ezzi G, Sitnicka EW, Jacobsen SE, Wakkach A, Blin-Wakkach C. Osteoclasts promote the formation of hematopoietic stem cell niches in the bone marrow. Journal of Experimental Medicine. 2012;209(3): 537-549.

[88] Nakamura T, Imai Y, Matsumoto T, Sato S, Takeuchi K, Igarashi K, et al. Estrogen prevents bone loss via estrogen receptor alpha and induction of Fas ligand in osteoclasts. Cell. 2007;130(5): 811-823.

[89] Oursler MJ, Landers JP, Riggs BL, Spelsberg TC. Oestrogen effects on osteoblasts and osteoclasts. Ann Med. 1993;25(4):361-371.

[90] Oursler MJ, Osdoby P, Pyfferoen J, Riggs BL, Spelsberg TC. Avian osteoclasts as estrogen target cells. Proc Natl Acad Sci U S A. 1991;88(15): 6613-6617.

[91] Oursler MJ, Pederson L, Pyfferoen J, Osdoby P, Fitzpatrick L, Spelsberg TC. Estrogen modulation of avian osteoclast lysosomal gene expression. Endocrinology. 1993;132(3):1373-1380.

[92] Kovacic N, Lukic IK, Grcevic D, Katavic V, Croucher P, Marusic A. The Fas/Fas ligand system inhibits differentiation of murine osteoblasts but has a limited role in osteoblast and osteoclast apoptosis. J Immunol. 2007;178(6):3379-3389.

[93] Krum SA, Miranda-Carboni GA, Hauschka PV, Carroll JS, Lane TF, Freedman LP, et al. Estrogen protects bone by inducing Fas ligand in osteoblasts to regulate osteoclast survival. EMBO J. 2008;27(3): 535-545.

[94] Vanderschueren D, Gaytant J, Boonen S, Venken K. Androgens and bone. Curr Opin Endocrinol Diabetes Obes. 2008;15(3):250-254.

[95] Weitzmann MN. Bone and the Immune System. Toxicol Pathol. 2017;45(7):911-924.

[96] Horvathova M, Ilavska S, Stefikova K, Szabova M, Krivosikova Z, Jahnova E, et al. The Cell Surface Markers Expression in Postmenopausal Women and Relation to Obesity and Bone Status. Int J Environ Res Public Health. 2017;14(7).

[97] Pacifici R, Rifas L, McCracken R, Avioli LV. The role of interleukin-1 in postmenopausal bone loss. Exp Gerontol. 1990;25(3-4):309-316.

[98] Cenci S, Toraldo G, Weitzmann MN, Roggia C, Gao Y, Qian WP, et al. Estrogen deficiency induces bone loss by increasing T cell proliferation and lifespan through IFN-gamma-induced class II transactivator. Proc Natl Acad Sci U S A. 2003;100(18):10405-10410.

[99] Cenci S, Weitzmann MN, Roggia C, Namba N, Novack D, Woodring J, et al. Estrogen deficiency induces bone loss by enhancing T-cell production of TNF-alpha. J Clin Invest. 2000;106(10): 1229-1237.

[100] Roggia C, Gao Y, Cenci S, Weitzmann MN, Toraldo G, Isaia G, et al. Up-regulation of TNF-producing T cells in the bone marrow: a key mechanism by which estrogen deficiency induces bone loss in vivo. Proc Natl Acad Sci U S A. 2001;98(24): 13960-13965.

[101] Roggia C, Tamone C, Cenci S, Pacifici R, Isaia GC. Role of TNF-alpha producing T-cells in bone loss induced by estrogen deficiency. Minerva Med. 2004;95(2):125-132.

[102] Weitzmann MN, Pacifici R. Estrogen deficiency and bone loss: an inflammatory tale. J Clin Invest. 2006;116(5):1186-1194.

[103] Kimble RB, Bain S, Pacifici R. The functional block of TNF but not of IL-6 prevents bone loss in ovariectomized mice. Journal of Bone and Mineral Research. 1997;12(6):935-941.

[104] Deselm CJ, Takahata Y, Warren J, Chappel JC, Khan T, Li X, et al. IL-17 mediates estrogen-deficient osteoporosis in an Act1-dependent manner. J Cell Biochem. 2012;113(9):2895-2902.

[105] Takayanagi H, Sato K, Takaoka A, Taniguchi T. Interplay between interferon and other cytokine systems in bone metabolism. Immunol Rev. 2005;208:181-193.

[106] Duque G, Huang DC, Dion N, Macoritto M, Rivas D, Li W, et al. Interferon-γ plays a role in bone formation in vivo and rescues osteoporosis in ovariectomized mice. Journal of Bone and Mineral Research. 2011;26(7):1472-1483.

[107] Osta B, Benedetti G, Miossec P. Classical and Paradoxical Effects of TNF-α on Bone Homeostasis. Frontiers in Immunology. 2014;5(48).

[108] Tyagi AM, Mansoori MN, Srivastava K, Khan MP, Kureel J, Dixit M, et al. Enhanced immunoprotective effects by anti-IL-17 antibody translates to improved skeletal parameters under estrogen deficiency compared with anti-RANKL and anti-TNF-α antibodies. J Bone Miner Res. 2014;29(9):1981-1992.

[109] Ginaldi L, De Martinis M, Ciccarelli F, Saitta S, Imbesi S, Mannucci C, et al. Increased levels of interleukin 31 (IL-31) in osteoporosis. BMC Immunology. 2015;16(1):60.

[110] Du D, Zhou Z, Zhu L, Hu X, Lu J, Shi C, et al. TNF-alpha suppresses osteogenic differentiation of MSCs by accelerating P2Y2 receptor in estrogen-deficiency induced osteoporosis. Bone. 2018;117:161-170.

[111] Cline-Smith A, Axelbaum A, Shashkova E, Chakraborty M, Sanford J, Panesar P, et al. Ovariectomy activates chronic low-grade inflammation mediated by memory T-cells which promotes osteoporosis in mice. J Bone Miner Res. 2020.

[112] Hodsman AB, Bauer DC, Dempster DW, Dian L, Hanley DA, Harris ST, et al. Parathyroid hormone and teriparatide for the treatment of osteoporosis: a review of the evidence and suggested guidelines for its use. Endocrine reviews. 2005;26(5):688-703.

[113] Lim SY, Bolster MB. Profile of romosozumab and its potential in the management of osteoporosis. Drug design, development and therapy. 2017;11:1221.

[114] Fixen C, Tunoa J. Romosozumab: a Review of Efficacy, Safety, and Cardiovascular Risk. Curr Osteoporos Rep. 2021.

[115] Saag KG, Zanchetta JR, Devogelaer JP, Adler RA, Eastell R, See K, et al. Effects of teriparatide versus alendronate for treating glucocorticoid-induced osteoporosis: thirty-six-month results of a randomized, double-blind, controlled trial. Arthritis Rheum. 2009;60(11):3346-3355.

[116] Tashjian AH, Jr., Gagel RF. Teriparatide [human PTH(1-34)]: 2.5 years of experience on the use and safety of the drug for the treatment of osteoporosis. J Bone Miner Res. 2006;21(3):354-365.

[117] Brandenburg VM, Verhulst A, Babler A, D'Haese PC, Evenepoel P, Kaesler N. Sclerostin in chronic kidney disease-mineral bone disorder think first before you block it! Nephrol Dial Transplant. 2019;34(3):408-414.

[118] Cosman F, Nieves JW, Dempster DW. Treatment sequence matters: anabolic and antiresorptive therapy for osteoporosis. Journal of bone and mineral research. 2017;32(2):198-202.

[119] Fink HA, MacDonald R, Forte ML, Rosebush CE, Ensrud KE, Schousboe JT, et al. Long-Term Drug Therapy and Drug Holidays for Osteoporosis Fracture Prevention: A Systematic Review. AHRQ Comparative Effectiveness Reviews. Rockville (MD)2019.

[120] Chong WP, Mattapallil MJ, Raychaudhuri K, Bing SJ, Wu S, Zhong Y, et al. The Cytokine IL-17A Limits Th17 Pathogenicity via a Negative Feedback Loop Driven by Autocrine Induction of IL-24. Immunity. 2020.

[121] Buchwald ZS, Kiesel JR, DiPaolo R, Pagadala MS, Aurora R. Osteoclast Activated FoxP3+ CD8+ T-Cells Suppress Bone Resorption in vitro. PLoS ONE. 2012;7(6):e38199–e38112.

[122] Buchwald ZS, Yang C, Nellore S, Shashkova EV, Davis JL, Cline A, et al. A Bone Anabolic Effect of RANKL in a Murine Model of Osteoporosis Mediated Through FoxP3 +CD8 T Cells. Journal of Bone and Mineral Research. 2015;30(8):1508-1522.

[123] Buchwald ZS, Aurora R. Osteoclasts and CD8 T Cells Form a Negative Feedback Loop That Contributes to Homeostasis of Both the Skeletal and Immune Systems. Clin Dev Immunol. 2013;2013. Article ID 429373.

[124] Buchwald ZS, Kiesel J, Yang C, DiPaolo R, Novack D, Aurora R. Osteoclast-induced Foxp3+ CD8 T-Cells Limit Bone Loss in Mice. Bone. 2013;56:163-173.

[125] Cline-Smith A, Gibbs J, Shashkova E, Buchwald ZS, Aurora R. Pulsed low-dose RANKL as a potential therapeutic for postmenopausal osteoporosis. JCI Insight. 2016;1(13):433-412.

Chapter 5

Bone Quality of the Dento-Maxillofacial Complex and Osteoporosis. Opportunistic Radiographic Interpretation

Plauto Christopher Aranha Watanabe,

Giovani Antonio Rodrigues, Marcelo Rodrigues Azenha,

Michel Campos Ribeiro, Enéas de Almeida Souza Filho,

Rafael Angelo Soares Vieira and Fabio Santos Bottacin

Abstract

Research suggests the use of different indexes on panoramic radiography as a way to assess BMD and to be able to detect changes in bone metabolism before fractures occur. Therefore, the objective of this chapter is to describe the use of these parameters as an auxiliary mechanism in the detection of low bone mineral density, as well as to characterize the radiographic findings of patients with osteoporosis.

Keywords: osteoporosis, oral cavity, panoramic radiography, mineral density of bone tissue, fractal dimension

1. Introduction

Osteoporosis is a chronic disease that affects the mineral density of bone tissue (BMD), leaving it more fragile and predisposing its carriers to a higher risk of fractures. The gold standard for the diagnosis of osteoporosis is dual X-ray densitometry (DXA), an exam that is difficult to access in some countries worldwide. Over the years, researchers have dedicated themselves to studying the radiographic findings of osteoporosis in gnathic bones in an attempt to create indexes or patterns that could assess BMD and thereby detect changes in bone metabolism before fractures occur. Thus, the objective of this chapter is to present concisely data on osteoporosis and to deepen themes related to the presence of the disease in the maxillomandibular region, as well as to review the literature presenting recent research on the use of imaging tests (X-rays, beam computed tomography, among others) to identify and aid in the diagnosis of osteoporosis [1].

2. Osteoporosis

Osteo Metabolic diseases are a set of disorders that affect the metabolism of bone tissue promoting a decrease in its mass and consequently causing bone fragility and an increased incidence of fractures. The various types of osteoporosis, rickets, osteomalacia, primary hyperparathyroidism and Paget's disease are the main diseases that affect the bones [2–4].

These disorders are characterized by an imbalance between the formation and remodeling of bone tissue and among the diseases belonging to this group the most prevalent is osteoporosis which affects bone microarchitecture resulting in tissue fragility and in most cases leading to fractures in various locations in the skeleton such as the spine, hip, femur and wrist [5].

Many factors contribute to the development of this condition, such as age, sex and ethnicity, which are among the main determinants of bone mass level and risk of fractures, and the clinical complications of the disease also include chronic pain, depression, deformities, loss of independence and increased mortality [6].

In operational and diagnostic terms, the World Health Organization (WHO) defines osteoporosis as a condition in which bone mineral density is equal to or less than 2.5 standard deviations below the peak of bone mass found in young adults. Currently, the diagnosis of osteoporosis is based on the identification of different risk factors, the most important of which is the low bone mineral density (BMD) of the femur and lumbar spine [7–10].

Although dual-beam X-ray densitometry (DXA) is considered the gold standard for the diagnosis of osteoporosis, its low predictive power and low availability make it impossible to use it as a method of population screening. The imbalance of bone metabolism caused by osteoporosis leads to a decrease in bone mineral throughout the body. Like other bones in the body, the jaw can be affected by systemic diseases or drug treatments even though it is not directly involved with the disease [7, 11].

3. Epidemiology

The number of osteoporosis cases in the United States of America (USA) was estimated at 14 million people in 2020, with more than two million bone fractures occurring annually as a result of osteoporosis, especially affecting women who account for 70% of cases. In men, although less prevalent, it is estimated that 30% of all hip fractures occur in this gender and the mortality rate due to the consequences of osteoporosis is higher in men than in women [1, 12].

In Brazil, South America, the statistics on the prevalence of osteoporosis are uncertain, showing great variations due to the size of the sample, the population studied and the methodologies employed. More recent studies, however, indicate that the projection for the next 5 years is that approximately 4,485,352 bone fractures will occur as a result of osteoporosis in Brazil, Mexico, Colombia and Argentina [6, 13–14].

As a result, it is relevant to study and deepen knowledge on this disease, which affects a large part of the world population and causes a high rate of morbidity and mortality, with approximately 20% of individuals who suffered hip fractures evolving to death one year after fracture. In Brazil, this rate is 23.6% of people who die 3 months after a fracture of the femur [15].

4. Diagnosis and treatment

The diagnosis of osteoporosis is made by examining bone densitometry (DXA) in which there will be a quantification of bone mineral density and from which it is possible to predict the risk of fractures. This exam method is technical-dependent. Other routine and radiological exams may also be required for this diagnosis and the evaluation of bone remodeling markers has been shown to be an important tool for clinical monitoring of patients undergoing drug treatment for osteoporosis [1].

Physical exercises with professional supervision are indicated for the non-pharmacological treatment of osteoporosis or osteopenia, as well as calcium and vitamin D supplementation are important and can be part of the treatment routine. In more severe cases, usually patients with a history of recent fractures or patients with a DXA T-score less than or equal to-2.5 standard deviations, pharmacological treatment is indicated [7].

5. Osteoporosis and oral cavity

Over time and the physiological aging process, maxillofacial structures also suffer from this action and especially the bones of the jaw and maxilla, as well as the dental cementum end up showing decreased vascularization, reduced metabolic capacity and in patients affected by osteoporosis, the decrease in bone mineral density can also affect the stomatognathic system [16].

When this occurs, the main oral manifestations of osteoporosis are related to the reduction of the alveolar ridge, increased porosity of the mandible and maxilla bone, periodontal changes, greater spacing between the bone trabeculae and the decrease in the maxillary bone mass and density. In addition to the aforementioned descriptions, researchers from the University of São Paulo (Dentistry Faculties of Ribeirão Preto and São Paulo) also highlight the changes that can occur in the temporomandibular joint, that is, through the reabsorption of its components, such as the condylar region. In addition to these changes in the TMJ, a greater contrast of the oblique line of the mandible and the cortical portion of the cervical verte-brae (frame aspect) can be seen in imaging studies and can contribute to the early recognition of systemic osteoporosis [16].

Thus, imaging tests are recommended to assess the involvement of the maxilla and mandible by osteoporosis, with panoramic radiography being the most used instrument for this purpose. This exam method is also technical-dependent, but regarding the main methods of analysis of bone quality that has been proposed by researchers, the radiomorphometric indices, has good accuracy, as it is also an orthopantomographic technique as we will see below.

6. Osteoporosis and periodontal disease

Tzu-Hsien L; et al. studied Association Between Periodontal Disease and Osteoporosis by Gender, being the diagnosis of periodontitis was defined on the basis of subgingival curettage, periodontal flap operation, and gingivectomy. They claim they found a significant association between periodontitis and osteoporosis among women (odds ratio: 1.96; 95% confidence interval 1.17–3.26) [17].

Regi et al., 2019 studied the radiographic comparison of mandibular bone quality in patients with chronic generalized periodontitis to assess osteoporosis of different age groups (60 patients), group 1 included patients in the age group of 30–44 years and group 2 with an age range of 45–60 years, using radio morpho-metric indices such as mandibular cortical index (MCI), mental index (MI), and panoramic mandibular index (PMI) in Indian population from dental panoramic radiographs. The authors could conclude that radiomorphometric indices could be used by general dentists to detect patients at higher risk of osteoporosis. This results are in agreement with Kalinowski et al, 2019 that studied the Correlations between periodontal disease, mandibular inferior cortex index and the osteoporotic fracture probability assessed by means of the fracture risk assessment body mass index tool (Inferior Cortex (MIC) index and osteoporotic fracture probability based on the FRAX BMI tool) [18].

This FRAX BMI tool with radiological evaluation of periodontal disease severity and MIC index could be used in dental practice in determining individual risk of osteoporotic fracture in females and provide new opportunities of selecting those potentially more prone to such fractures. Years before, Iwasaki et al., 2013 conducted cross-sectional study to evaluate the possible association between BMD and clinical attachment loss (AL) with dental restoration information in Japanese community-dwelling postmenopausal females (397 females (average age: 68.2 years). The results of this study indicated that low systemic BMD was associated with severe AL in Japanese community-dwelling postmenopausal females. Jonasson and Rythén, 2016, had already evaluated alveolar bone loss in osteoporosis. They rated that bone turnover rate in the alveolar mandibular process is probably the fastest; and thus, the first signs of osteoporosis could be revealed at the alveolar bone [19].

Still According to these authors, sparse trabeculation in the mandibular premolar region (large intertrabecular spaces and thin trabeculae) is a reliable sign of osteopenia and a high skeletal fracture risk. But, Springe and Soboleva at 2014 founded that postmenopausal women with reduced general BMD do not appear to have a reduction in the size of the mandibular residual ridge in contrast the results of the Al-Jabrah and Al-Shumailan, also 2014 that founded reduced mandibular height that would be directly related to age and duration of complete denture wearing and women are at more risk to have ridge resorption compared to men.

7. Principles of panoramic radiography

In 1948, Paatero at the University of Helsinki developed orthopantomography based on the principles of medical tomography, that is, a radiographic technique that allows the image of a section of the body to be widely used in medicine and after the advancement in implantology it started to be more used in dentistry. Thus, panoramic radiography is an extra-oral radiographic technique that is more suitable for allowing a better assessment of maxillary bones when compared to intraoral radiographs such as periapical, interproximal or bitewing radiography [20].

For panoramic radiography (PAN), the patient remains immobile while the X-ray source and radiographic sensors move in the opposite direction at one or more centers of rotation. These rotation points can be internal or external to the focal layer. Focal layer in tomography or "focal plane" or "image layer" is the plane that is not blurred in the radiographic image (**Figure 1**).

Panoramic radiography or pantomography is produced using the tomographic curve-surface and is performed by rotating a narrow beam of radiation in a horizontal plane around a virtual point/axis (called the center of rotation) positioned inside the oral cavity. Film and head move in the opposite direction around the patient, who remains stationary. Blurring is determined by the tube distance, focal plane distance, film distance and tube rotation orientation.

The center of rotation changes as the film/sensor and head rotate, allowing the image layer to adapt to the elliptical shape of the dental arches. With this, the vertical and horizontal dimensions are correlated only when the object is within a particular zone, or section plane that represents the image layer, best interpreted as the focal layer. This zone actually corresponds to a three-dimensional area in which the structures are reasonably focused or well defined. Thus, the positioning of the patient in the X-ray apparatus should be such that the dental arches are positioned strictly within this cutting area, resulting in a clear image of the teeth. That way,

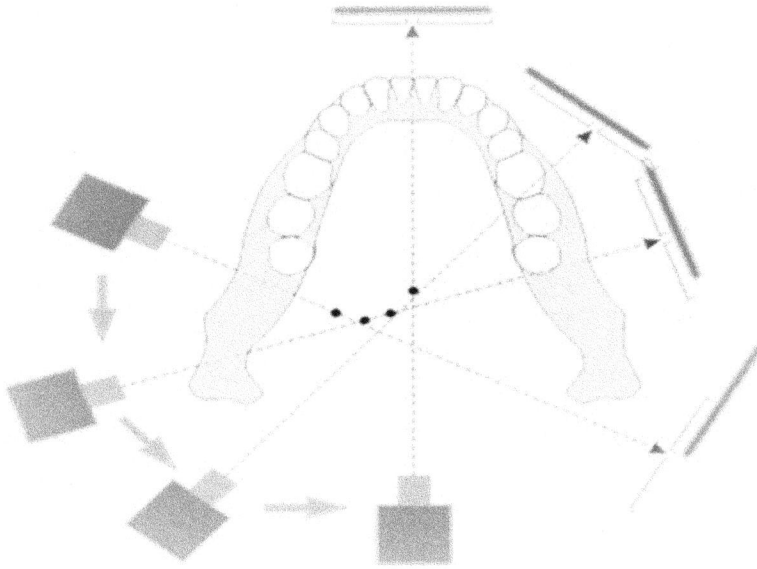

Figure 1.
Schematic illustrating the principle of panoramic radiography (PAN).

each manufacturer of panoramic X-ray apparatus recommends different layers of cut, because, of course, the dental arches are very different around the world. Objects outside the focal layer, distort. The best equipment allows you to focus on the most different dental arches, always in maximum detail (**Figure 2**) [21].

For the interpretation of these radiographic images, some characteristics need to be considered: objects closer to the film will be narrowed, objects closer to the tube will be widened and out of focus, objects located through the buccal teeth will

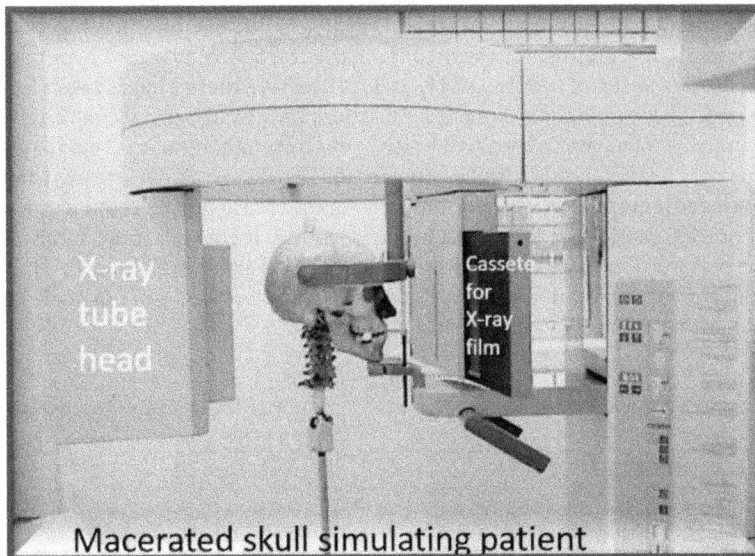

Figure 2.
Phantom, simulating the positioning of the patient in the panoramic X-ray equipment.

be projected inferiorly and objects located by lingual/palatal teeth will be projected higher. Objects located in the center of the cutting layer will be enlarged by a known factor, usually supplied by the equipment manufacturer, by about 25–40% [22].

Advantages of panoramic radiography:

- Features a unique dental exam through a panoramic representation of the stomatognathic system, including ATM, styloid processes and maxillary sinuses

- Allows the detection of the functional and pathological relationship and its effects on the stomatognathic system

- Provides a document for the treatment and preservation plan

- Reduces radiation exposure through a strategic rotational system that covers a large area

Disadvantages of panoramic radiography:

- Patients with extreme class II and III dental relationships make it impossible to have optimal images of the anterior teeth segments

- The ratio of the focus-object distance to the object-film distance is not identical in all cases, which results in a constant magnification factor

- Accurate measures are questioned

- Structures that reside outside the focus layer can be superimposed on normal structures of the jaw and simulate a pathology

The "Guidelines for the Selection of Patients for Dental Radiographic Examinations", prepared in 2004, by a panel of experts from the American Dental Association-ADA, recommends panoramic radiographic examination together with interproximal radiographs, for every initial patient who needs state assessment. General of the teeth and mouth, and that does not have these images taken in the near period. These guidelines are not a substitute for initial clinical examination and anamnesis. The patient's vulnerability to environmental factors that may affect his or her oral health should also be considered. The Expert Panel stresses that the panoramic radiographic examination has the main advantages of reducing the dose of radiation exposure, at a lower cost and in addition, it covers a much larger area than the periapical radiographic examination (**Tables 1** and **2; Figure 3**).

In addition to this main indication, panoramic radiographs will normally be indicated in situations where (**Table 2** and **Figure 4**):

New patient - child with mixed dentition	Periapical / occlusal and interproximal or panoramic
New patient - Edentulous	Whole or panoramic mouth
Growth and development assessment - mixed dentition	Periapical / occlusal or panoramic
Growth and development assessment - permanent dentition	Periapical or panoramic to evaluate 3Ms

Table 1.
Types of requests for different patients and the radiographic prescription indicated.

	Teeth region on panoramic radiography. Teeth are the main focus of analysis for dentists.
	Region of the jaws and mandible on panoramic radiography. In these regions we will focus the analysis on the maxillary sinuses, their relationship with the dental roots, nasal fossa (septum and lower nasal turbinates) m, in addition to the mandibular body, mandibular canal, mental foramen and lower mandibular cortex, in general, very focused these panoramic images.
	Region of mandibular branches on panoramic radiography. We can also analyze styloid apophysis and possible calcifications of the hyoid style ligament, in addition to the initial third of the cervical spine in many images, mainly of older people.
	Region of the mandibular heads, where in general we can make a comparison between both, and the region of the hyoid bones (double image). Where, just above this region is the bifurcation of the carotid artery where in many situations we can suspect images compatible with atheromas, except for the images of the tritite / thyroid cartilage.

Table 2.
Panoramic radiography (pan) - ORTHOPANTOMOGRAPHY.

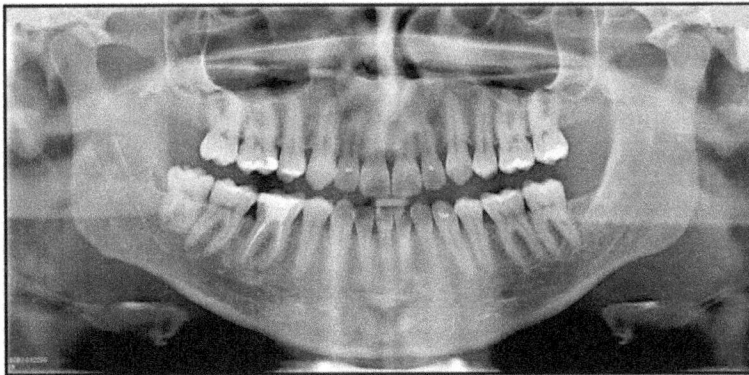

Figure 3.
Image of digital panoramic radiography.

1. A real suspicion, based on a clinical examination, of extensive and / or active pathology outside the alveolar bone.

2. Problems with symptomatic third molars, where the likely treatment will be followed.

3. Evaluation for placement of dental implants

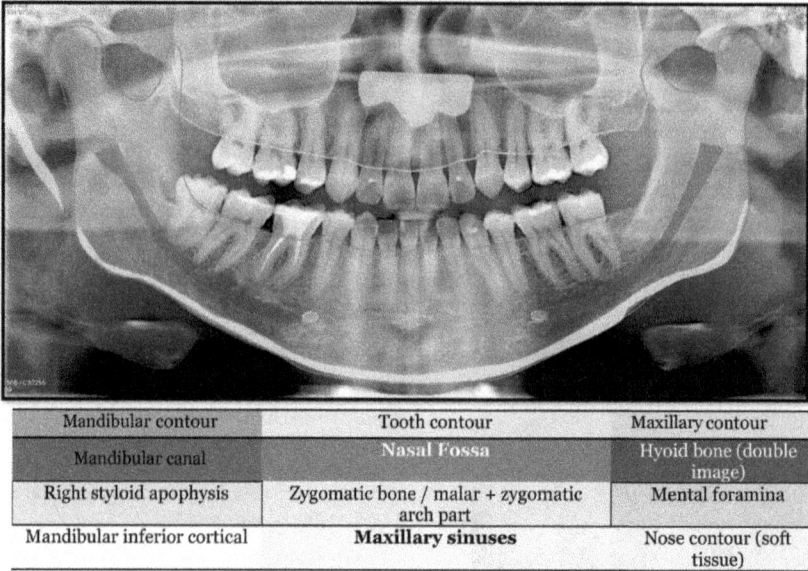

Mandibular contour	Tooth contour	Maxillary contour
Mandibular canal	**Nasal Fossa**	Hyoid bone (double image)
Right styloid apophysis	Zygomatic bone / malar + zygomatic arch part	Mental foramina
Mandibular inferior cortical	**Maxillary sinuses**	Nose contour (soft tissue)

Figure 4.
Anatomical structures on panoramic radiography.

4. Trauma involving more than one tooth or suspected of underlying bone damage.

5. Periodontal participation involving a generalized "bag" of more than 5 mm, where the equivalent diagnostic information would require more than 3 intraoral radiographs.

6. Multiple extractions, where equivalent diagnostic information would require more than 3 intraoral radiographs.

7. Evaluation of the growth and development of the maxillomandibular complex for orthodontics/orthopedics and orthognathic surgery.

Below you can see the main regions of the panoramic radiography (**Table 2**), as well as the anatomical structures in **Figure 4.**

8. Radiomorphometric indices in osteoporosis

The human skeleton can be divided into axial spine, head on the central axis of the body, and appendicular to the limbs, arms and legs. For medicine, the main structures studied refer to the spine and head of the femur in the hip, and forearm, as these offer the possibility of fractures. We can assume that the maxillomandibular complex is in the head, and thus, it would have characteristics similar to the spine. This really happens, but mainly with the maxilla. The mandible has unique characteristics, even being part of the axial skeleton. Studies show that the decrease in bone mineral density affects the morphometric, densitometric and architectural properties mandible in osteoporotic patients on radiographs, and the main radiographic signs of this condition include a relative generalized radiolucency of the maxilla and mandible or bone rarefaction, decreased thickness of the mandibular inferior cortex, added to erosions in that same cortex, in addition to generalized accentuation or cortical, maxillary sinus, mandibular canal, nasal fossa, oblique line, among others (**Figures 5–8**) [23].

Several radiomorphometric indices have been proposed to assess the correlation of loss of bone mineral density in the mandible with DXA as the thickness of the mandibular cortex, the mandibular panoramic index, the alveolar crest resorption index, the mandibular cortical index and the fractal dimension of the alveolar/basal bone. These indices represent variations in bone morphology and may be associated with systemic factors [24].

The main measures referring to the radiomorphometric indices relate to the mandible, and as we saw above, in the description of the panoramic radiographic technique, it must always be in the cut layer or cut plane to obtain panoramic radiographs, and so, in general, they are focused. As we have seen, it is also common to produce enlargement of anatomical structures in these panoramic images, and this is provided by the manufacturer of X-ray equipment, on average, but it will hardly vary from structure to structure in different patients. We also know that there are different magnifications between the X-ray equipment, but they all provide the average magnification. Therefore, starting from the

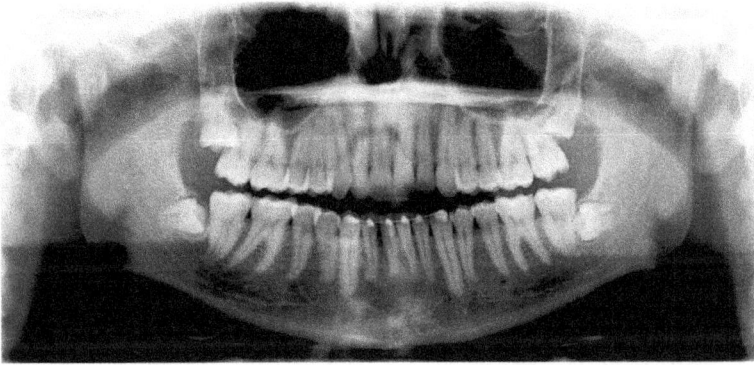

Figure 5.
Panoramic radiograph of a young adult patient, 21 years old. Note the characteristics of the bony trabeculae, lower cortical mandible (including thickness), region of the retromolar trigone.

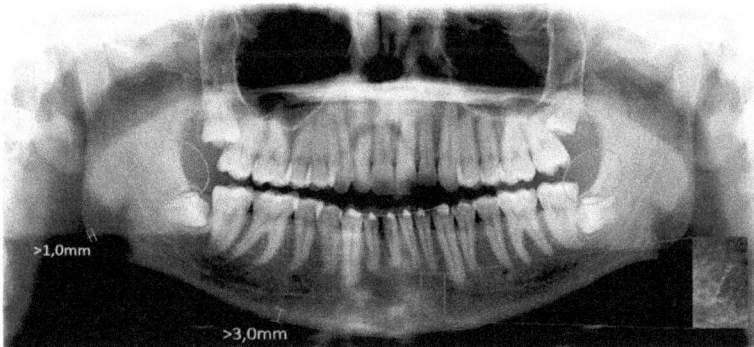

Figure 6.
Panoramic radiograph of a 21-year-old male adult patient. Note the measurements taken at the mandibular angle (goniac index), still at the mandibular inferior cortex, at the height of the mental foramen (mental index), Look at region of the retromolar trigone, the characteristics of the mandibular bone trabeculae (highlighted), in basal bone.

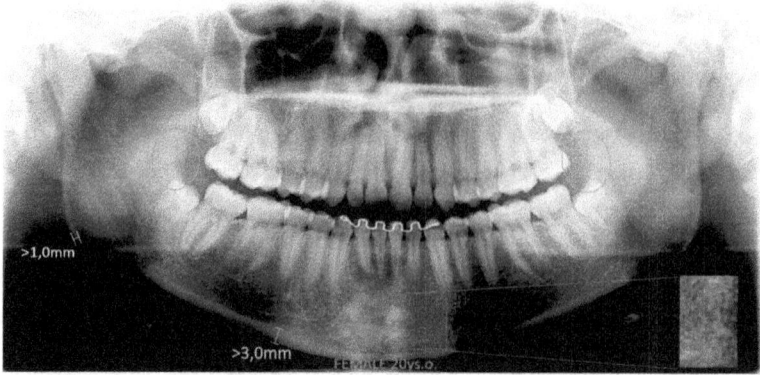

Figure 7.
Panoramic radiograph of a 21-year-old female adult patient. Note the measurements taken at the mandibular angle (goniac index), still at the mandibular inferior cortex, at the height of the mental foramen (mental index), Look at region of the retromolar trigone, the characteristics of the mandibular bone trabeculae (highlighted), in basal bone.

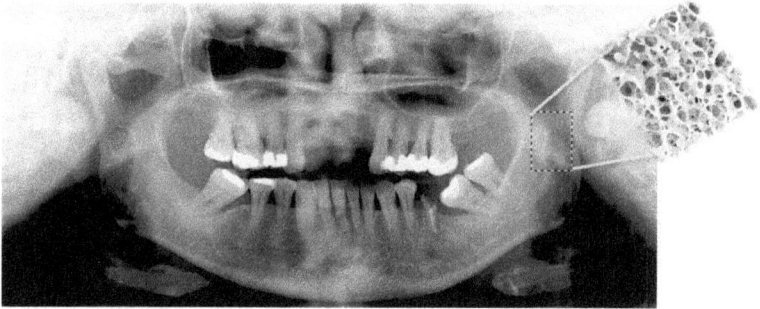

Figure 8.
Panoramic radiograph of a young adult male patient, 41 years old. This patient has initial periodontal disease. Note the characteristics of the bone trabeculae in the mandibular ramus (highlighted), a region free of occlusal forces from dental elements.

premise that we will only analyze images with excellent quality, that is, with the mandible fully contained in the cutting plane of the X-ray equipment, that is, focused, we can rather rely on these measures related to the radiomorphometric indices [25].

The Klemetti index, also called the mandibular cortical index (ICM), was introduced in 1994, based on a sample of postmenopausal women with osteoporosis and it is an index of bone quality morphological evaluation. This qualitative index, classifies the cortical mandibular zone located distal to the mental foramen in three categories: C1 (normal cortex) - when the endosteal margin of the cortex is regular and without defects on both sides; C2 (moderately eroded cortex) - the endosteal margin has semilunar defects or has cortical residues on one or both sides; C3 (severely eroded cortex) - the cortical layer clearly shows the existence of large residues and has a porous aspect [26–27].

Researchers have studied the usefulness of panoramic radiographs in the diagnosis of osteoporosis in the Korean population. In this study, 194 radiographs dated between 2007 and 2010 were analyzed. The authors used three panoramic indexes, the mental index, the mandibular cortical index and a visual estimation index for exam analysis. It is important to note that in this study, each observer was unaware of the results of each patient's DXA, nor access to their personal information, such as age and sex, as the authors understood that this could influence the final result. After analyzing the data, it is concluded that the three indexes investigated presented themselves as useful tools for the diagnosis of osteoporosis [28–29].

The mandibular cortical thickness index was the most useful as a high-risk exclusion method for a population with low levels of bone mineral density. In turn, the Klemetti index was considered a useful tool, since approximately 80% of people with moderate or severe erosion of the mandibular cortex have osteopenia. However, the risk of bias related to the subjectivity of a qualitative measure such as the Klemetti index needs to be taken into account. Furthermore, the authors suggest that further studies on this topic are needed in order to obtain more accurate and reliable results and conclusions [28].

Another important tool to measure bone quality is the Fractal Dimension, mainly in the evaluation of bone trabeculation, but it is also used in cortical analysis. By Fractal Dimension (FD) it is also possible to assess bone morphometric parameters such as trabecular area or connectivity on panoramic radiographs. Moreover, FD of trabecular bone has been associated with bone strength, according to Camargo et al., 2017 and concluded that FD and MCI offer a significant and relatively high sensitivity, whereas MCW offers a high specificity for screening low BMD. In 2016 these authors, Camargo et al., assessed the correlation between different quality analysis parameters of trabecular pattern in digital panoramic radiographs and relations with forearm bone mass density (BMD) performed by DXA by panoramic radiography. The analysis showed correlations with each other, detecting alterations in the trabecular pattern, significantly, however it cannot be related to BMD with FD. In 2018, Vijayalakshmi et al., studied clinically by estimating and comparing the measurement of trabecular bone pattern in the mandible of normal and osteoporotic volunteers. The authors did not show any significant difference in its architecture between normal and osteoporotic individuals as defined by BMD by periapical radiography. But recommended used these techniques using better-standardized resolution strategies and different estimation methods to gain more insight [30].

Kato CN, et al., 2020 reviewed the use of fractal analysis (FA) in dental images finding 78 articles were found in which FA was applied to panoramic radiographs (34), periapical radiographs (21), bitewing radiographs (4) and concluded that the FD are widely applied to the study of images at dentistry. In this same year, Bulut et al., studied the mandibular indexes and fractal properties on the panoramic radiographs of the patients using aromatase inhibitors (AI) to determine the mandibular cortical and trabecular bone changes in females with breast cancer. Concluded that AI use affects bone quality and evaluating FD and another mandibular index in panoramic radiography and FD can be used to determine the effect of this drug on the jaw bones in the early period [31–32].

Therefore, it appears that panoramic radiographs can be used as tools to detect low mineral bone density, not for the purpose of diagnosing a certain disease, but rather to identify and properly refer the patient for investigation by bone densitometry, for example, allowing to intercept the progress of the disease.

Despite the vast literature on the subject, there are still radiographic signs that have not been studied, such as the oblique line. It is relatively common to observe on radiographs, an enhancement of the oblique line due to the marked loss of trabecular bone mass in women over 65 years old and toothless, since there is an evident loss of trabecular bone mass in the jaw body and less loss of cortical. Other studies also indicate that the clear highlight of the oblique line and the cervical spine covering plates against the spongy part are signs of osteoporosis. In addition to radiographic signs, other analyzes were not used in osteoporosis, such as the evaluation of inter-trabecular angles to analyze the bone microarchitecture of the mandible [16].

Another important opportunity to study/observe bone sites affected by osteoporosis before as opportunistic dates. This can happen in several and bring, really, important analyzes. Pickhardt et al., 2013 proposed to study To evaluate abdominal computed tomography (CT)-derived bone mineral density (BMD) assessment compared with dual-energy x-ray absorptiometry (DXA) measures for identifying osteoporosis by using CT scans performed for other clinical indications. It was studied 1867 adults undergoing CT and DXA. CT-attenuation values (in Hounsfield units [HU]) of trabecular bone between the T12 and L5 vertebral levels. Thus, the authors were able to conclude that abdominal CT images that include the lumbar spine can be used to identify patients with osteoporosis or normal BMD without additional radiation exposure or cost. Already Buckens et al., 2015 performed opportunistic screening for osteoporosis using computed tomography (CT) examinations that happen to visualize the spine can be used to identify patients with osteoporosis. The authors sought to verify the diagnostic performance of vertebral Hounsfield unit (HU) measurements on routine CT examinations for diagnosing osteoporosis in a separate, external population. This population had CT examination of the chest or abdomen and had also received a dual energy X-ray absorptiometry (DXA) test were retrospectively included. CTs were evaluated for vertebral fractures and vertebral attenuation (density) values were measured. It was possible to verify that simple trabecular vertebral density measurements on routine CT contain diagnostic information related to bone mineral density, but with lower diagnostic accuracy than previously reported. Anyway the authors considered this information might be useful when considering the implementation of opportunistic osteoporosis screening. Also 2015, Barngkgei et al. investigated the use of cone beam computed tomography (CBCT) for predicting osteoporosis based on the cervical vertebrae CBCT-derived radiographic density (RD) using the CBCT-viewer program and concluded that CBCT-derived RD of cervical vertebrae can predict osteoporosis status.

In this line of thought, Cheade et al., 2018 and Cheade et al., 2019, correlated between the bone densities jaws and cervical spine through the HU scale measured in Multislice Computed Tomography (MCT), as opportunistic Screening for Osteoporosis. The authors concluded that there is a positive weak correlation between the cervical vertebrae and buccal sites, but moderate correlation of the

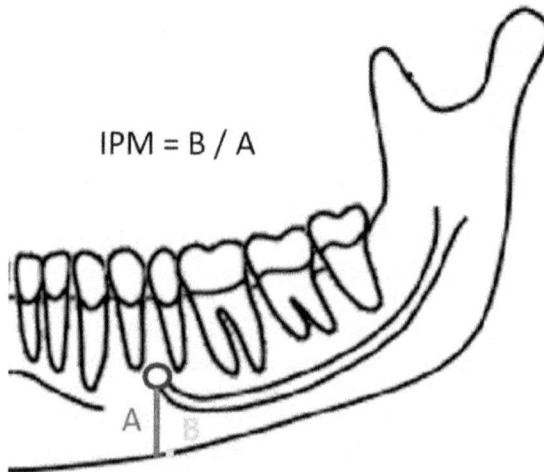

$$IPM = B / A$$

Figure 9.
Schematic drawing of the mandibular panoramic index.

cervical vertebrae with the anterior region of the maxilla was funded. Cheade et al., 2019, concluded in this study that as the HU values of the anterior and posterior mandible bone correlate with the HU values of the cervical bone, this test can be applied to osteoporosis screening tools [33–34].

Mandibular Panoramic Index (IPM): ratio of the thickness of the mandibular cortex, measured on a line perpendicular to the base of the mandible, at the height of the center of the mental foramen (A), by the distance between the lower limit of

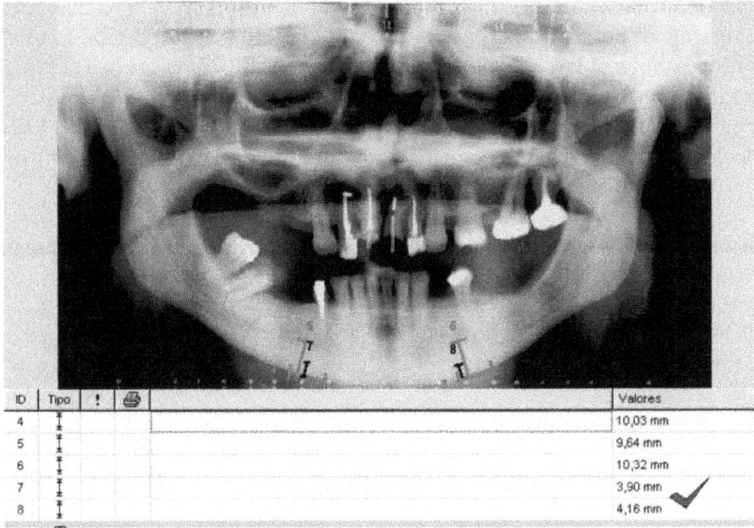

Figure 10.
Radiographic drawing of the mandibular panoramic index.

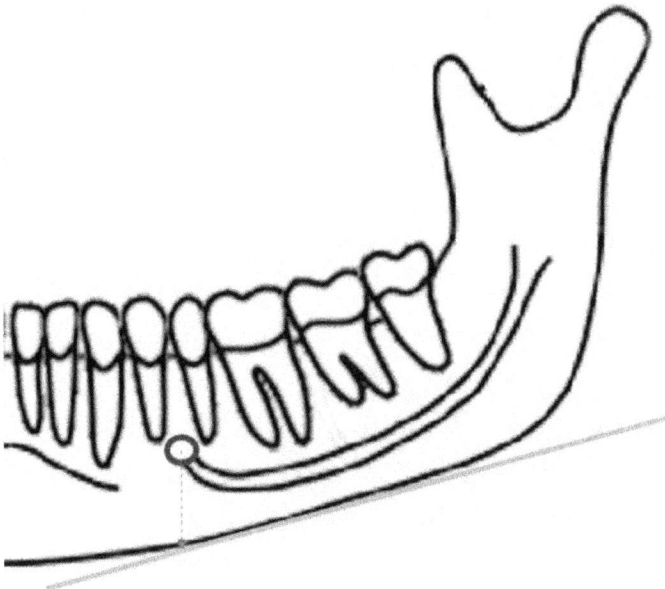

Figure 11.
Schematic drawing of the mentonian index.

the mandibular canal and the base of the mandible (B) having as reference value normal IPM greater than or equal to 0.3 (**Figures 9** and **10**) [27].

Mentonian Index (IM): the thickness of the mandibular cortex, measured on the line perpendicular to the base of the mandible (blue line), at the height of the center of the mental foramen (dashed line) will be considered as having a normal IM reference value greater or equal to 3.1 mm (**Figures 11** and **12**) [35].

Mandibular Cortical Index (ICM): the mandibular cortical is evaluated in a qualitative and visual way in three categories C1 (normal cortex) - when the endosteal margin of the cortex is regular and without defects on both sides; C2 (moderately eroded cortex) - the endosteal margin has semilunar defects or has cortical residues on one or both sides; C3 (severely eroded cortex) - the cortical layer clearly shows the existence of large residues and has a porous aspect (**Figure 13**) [36].

Fractal Dimension (FD): Digital radiographs are an increasingly popular option in the clinic nowadays. Digitally, such images are composed of pixels with a specific numerical value for each one, two principally methods are of evaluating the pixels

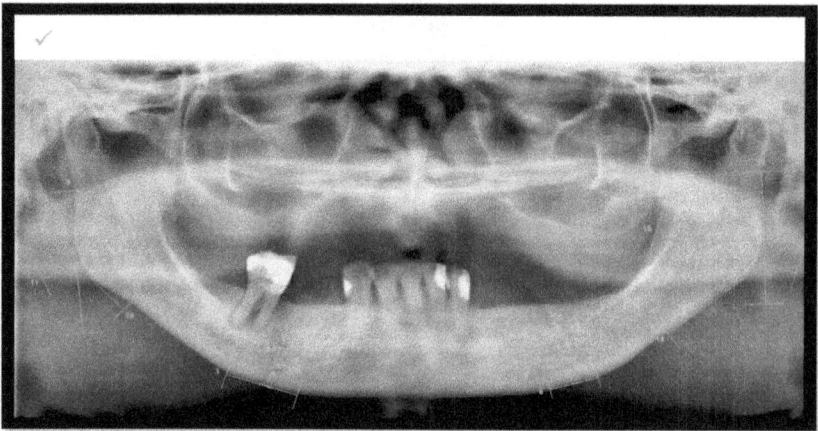

Figure 12.
Radiographic drawing of the mentual index and goniac index measured in mandibular angle.

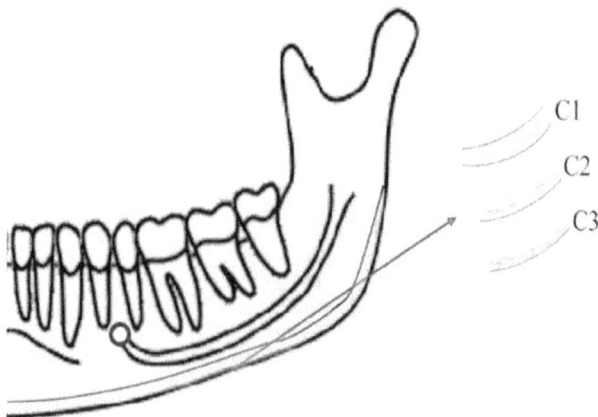

Figure 13.
Schematic drawing of the mandibular cortical index.

in these images: Fractal dimension (FD) and Pixel Intensity (PI) analyses. FD is expressed numerically and consists in describing complex shapes and structural patterns in the bone. PI is a grayscale measure, ranging from zero (black) to 256 (white) in a 8-bit digital image (Von Mulhen et al., 1999). Note in **Figure 16**, line A, image 47 has FD = 1.6038, and the% E.T. (percentage of trabecular structures) is equal to 11.28. Now notice line C, image 52, where the FD = 1.3686, and the% E.T. (percentage of trabecular structures) is equal to 5.61. The connectivity of image 47 is 6103.5 and of image 52, only 34.2 (**Figures 14–16**) [37].

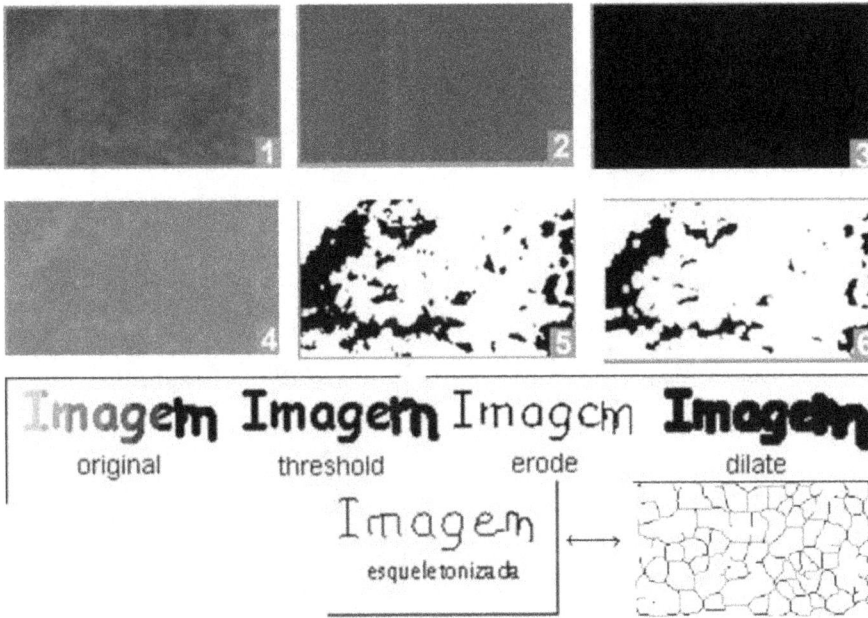

Figure 14.
*Step by step method of the fractal dimension and schematic drawing of the skeletonization process. 1, region of interest of trabecular bone from digitized radiograph of anterior maxilla. 2, highlighted ROI copy of the image in **Figure 7**, with "Gaussian blur" of 33 radius (pixels). 3. Result of subtracting **Image 1**, from **Image 2**. 4, result of adding 128. 5, result of binary transformation (threshold) of the **Image 4**, with 128 brightness value. 6, result of the erode process of the image **Image 5** above.*

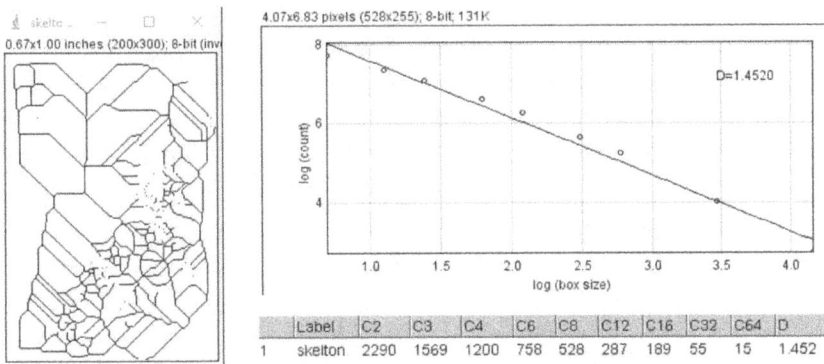

Figure 15.
*Graphic with the numerical result of the fractal dimension value (D = 1.4520) of the skeletonized image sample, seen on the right (ROI seen in **Figure 6**).*

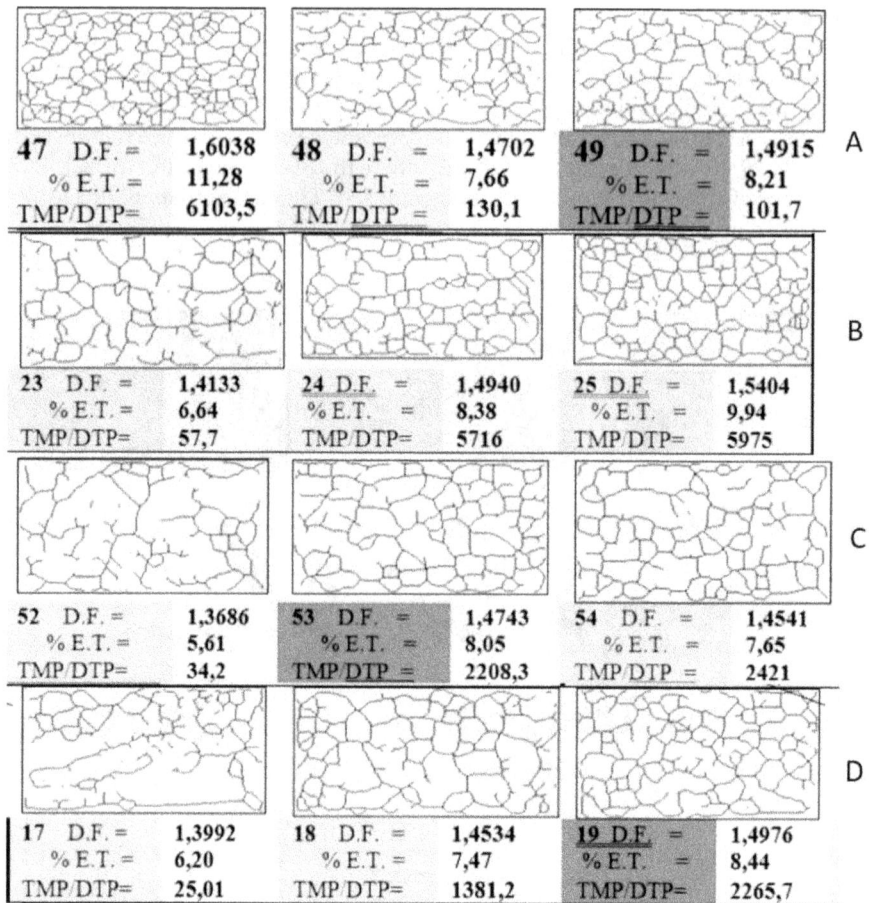

Figure 16.
Samples of skeletonized mandibular regions of interest with the respective fractal dimension values. These regions of interest would be implant sites (ROI similar to the one seen in **Figure 6**, *lying).*

9. Advances in research

In 1991 Benson studied 353 adult individuals between 30 and 79 years of age, equally separated by gender, ethnicity and age, described a measurement index on dental radiography which he called the mandibular index. In 1994, Klemetti compared the diagnostic efficacy of three panoramic indices in relation to bone mineral density in healthy and osteoporotic patients and indicated that panoramic radiography could not be used as a method for diagnosing osteoporosis, but that its indexes could be used to evaluate the disease in the gnathic bones [27].

Nakamoto et al., 2003 described the importance of detecting low bone mineral density in postmenopausal women as a way to reduce the incidence of osteoporosis fractures and justified that indices performed on panoramic radiography can be used as a means of detecting these women and tool to refer them for medical evaluation and DXA. As a result, panoramic radiography returns to the scene of science as a way to visualize changes in osteoporosis in the oral cavity and in a systematic way. This information was validated by Taguchi in 2004 and 2005 [38, 39].

In 2006, Yasar carried out a study whose objective was to evaluate the relationship between osteoporosis and the use of radiographic indexes in PAN. In this study, the introduction of the use of fractal dimension analysis in radiographic images began, however, it was concluded that only measurement of the thickness of the mandibular cortex obtained a statistical difference between the groups of healthy and osteoporotic patients. Later, in 2007, the OSTEODENT project, a collaboration between European research centers for the study of osteoporosis and oral cavity, validated the 2006 findings demonstrating that patients with mandibular cortical thickness less than 3 millimeters were referred for osteoporosis evaluation [40].

In the same year, Taguchi drew the attention of the scientific community to assess the risk of low bone density in the spine of postmenopausal patients who presented oral alterations in osteoporosis. In 2009, Watanabe found a correlation between the elongation of the styloid process and osteoporosis, in addition to also evaluating the radiographic images that indicated calcifications in the blood vessels and the presence of osteoporosis [41].

Continuing his studies, Taguchi in 2010 presented parameters for the evaluation and screening of patients in dental clinic for osteoporosis and again two indexes

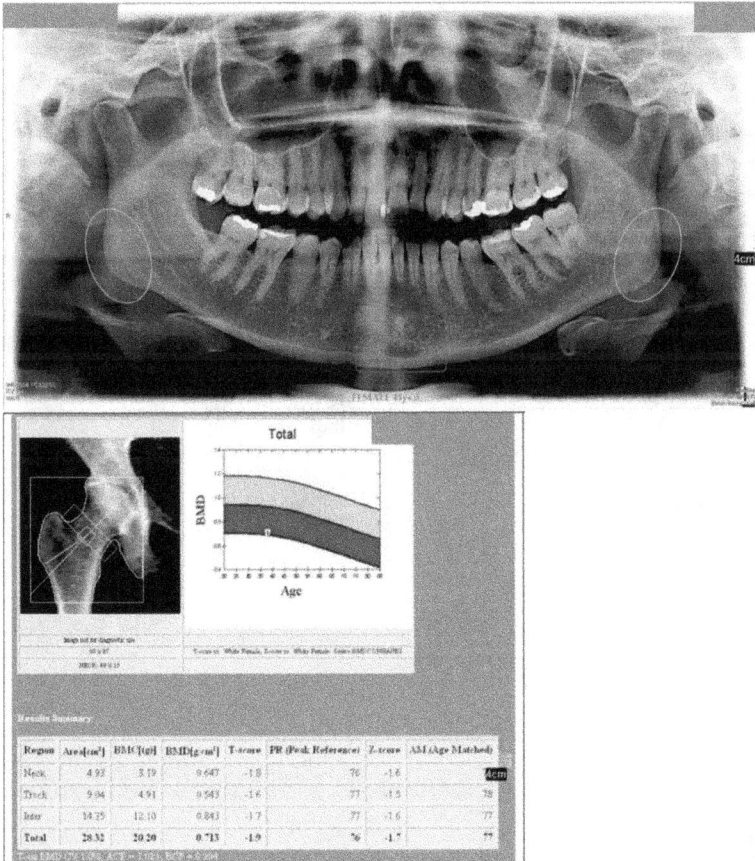

Figure 17.
Panoramic radiograph with some small bone quality details of a patient with a T-score pointing to OSTEOPENIA on the hip, or the head of the femur. Note the mandibular bone rarefaction. The mandibular inferior cortex is class II, according to Klemetti. Erosion is seen in the anterior region of the mandible, a region disregarded by Klemetti, as this author performed his classification on panoramic analog radiographs, on film, and at a time (1993–1994) when panoramic X-ray equipment had no technical development for better to focus on that region, and they still did not use digital images. The panoramic X-ray equipment had an excellent development since the 21st century, and thus, today we can even consider the anterior mandibular region for these analyzes. We also see that the lower cortex at the angle of the mandible on both sides has excess streaks, showing activity.

were discarded as predictors of osteoporosis by Leite et al., in the same year, being the indexes of the antegonial and gonial angles (look the **Figure 17**). So, in 2012 Kavitha started studies on digital panoramic radiographs and Devlin in 2013 did not rule out, through a systematic literature review, the use of DXA to the detriment of panoramic radiography [42–44].

Other studies became more popular and the researchers started to evaluate other diseases and conditions through indices in panoramic radiography, such as periodontal disease for example (look the reabsorption at **Figures 18** and **19**). In 2017, Munhoz et al., Also investigated the relationship between radiographic indexes, type 2 diabetes mellitus and osteoporosis and since then several studies have sought to define the use of digital tools in oral radiographs for different purposes [45].

Gomes et al., 2014 compared the assessment of mandibular indices on panoramic and cross sectional images using forty-four cone beam computed

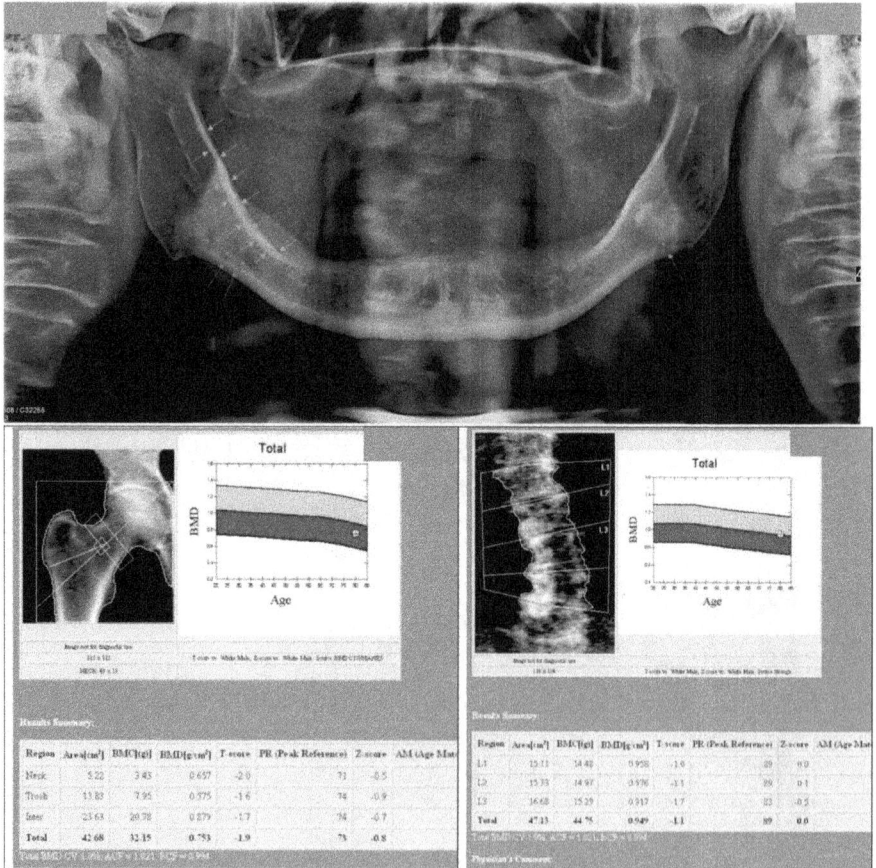

Figure 18.
Panoramic radiography with some small details in bone quality, of an edentulous patient, and with a T-score pointing to OSTEOPENIA in the hip, and in the spine. Note the mandibular bone rarefaction, which is more evident in the sharp contrast of the oblique line, in the region of the retromolar wheat on both sides. The oblique line is a mandibular reinforcement structure, but note its excessive brightness, or its sharp contrast, mainly due to the mandibular bone rarefaction, which causes this brightness to increase. The mandibular inferior cortex is class II, according to Klemetti, and the red arrows point to specific erosions in this structure. Another detail is the loss of the cortical or walls of the mandibular canals on both sides (pointed only on the left side). In addition, it is possible to see the frame aspect of the cervical vertebrae on both sides, indicating the substantial loss of trabecular bone, similar to the rarefaction of the mandibular body. Thus, it is possible to notice in the panoramic radiographic image a generalized cortical enhancement, showing the loss of trabecular structures as a whole.

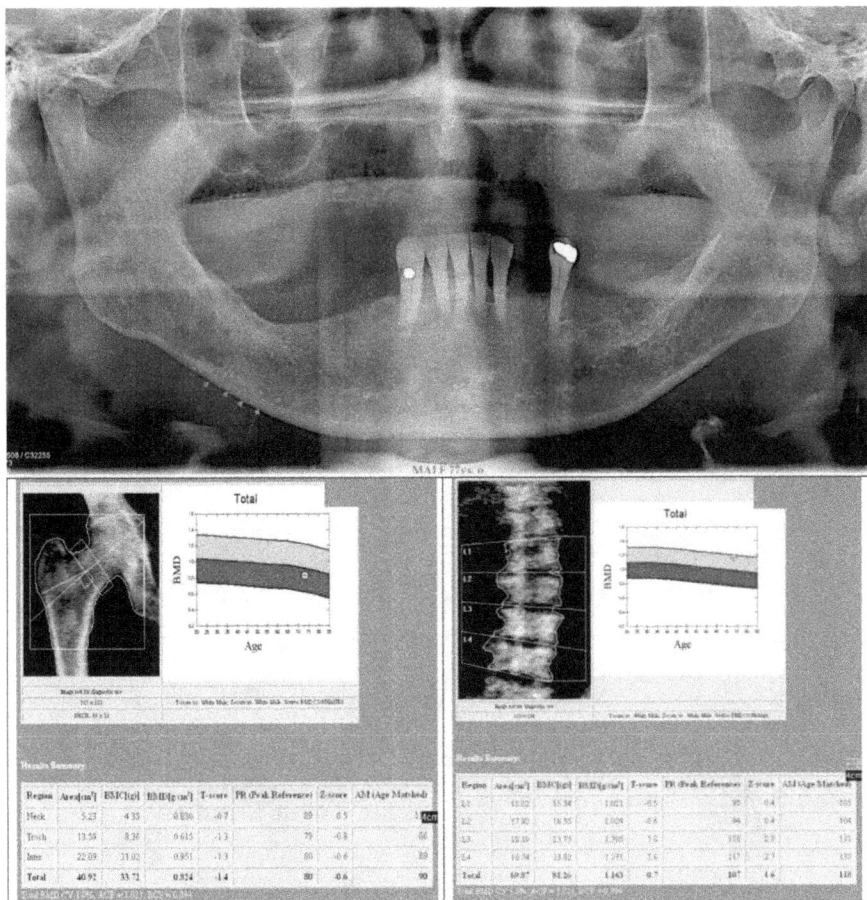

Figure 19.
Panoramic radiography with some small details in bone quality, of a partially edentulous patient, with only 6 teeth in the mandible, with a T-score pointing to OSTEOPENIA in the hip, and normality in the spine. The spine, an axial site, as we know, is more trabecular. The femur site would be more cortical. The red arrows point to several erosions in the mandibular inferior cortical on the right side, typically classifying this cortical as Klemetti class II-III. However, the left side cortex is still more preserved. However, we also see that the corticals of the mandibular canal on both sides cannot be delineated or are disappearing. . This patient has evident periodontal disease, with widespread alveolar bone crest resorption.

tomography (CBCT) images from postmenopausal female subjects aged more than 45 years without systemic changes. The appearance of the inferior cortex of the mandible was classified according to the mandibular index: C1, the endosteal margin of the cortex was even and sharp; C2, the endosteal margin presented semilunar defects or appeared to form endosteal cortical residues; or C3, the cortical layer formed heavy endosteal cortical residues and was clearly porous [46].

The authors found no statistically significant difference between the exams and concluded that the mandibular index assigned in tomographic images is comparable to that obtained in panoramic images, what was expected, since we were dealing with patients without systemic changes, understand, without an apparent risk of osteoporosis, and we must also consider that the mandibular inferior cortex, as a rule, must be in the focal layer of the panoramic radiographic image, the which favors this analysis of the Klemetti classification (**Figure 19**). This similar results was found by Cal Alonso, 2016, at panoramic radiography and CBCT panoramic reconstruction, but the higher values found for the cross-sectional slices certainly would be associated with better accuracy assessment for the CBCT images [47].

Van Dessel et al., also in 2016, study the quantification of bone quality using different cone beam computed tomography devices in comparison to multi-slice computed tomography (MSCT) and micro computed tomography (micro-CT) for objectively assessing cortical bone quality prior to implant placement and trabecular bone, but edentulous human mandibular bone samples (look the **Figures 18** and **19**. This authors found high resolution CBCT offers as a clinical alternative to MSCT to objectively determine the bone quality prior to implant placement. However, not all tested CBCT machines have sufficient resolution to accurately depict the network or cortical bone. Kenawy et al., 2017, conducted a study aimed to assess the effectiveness of radiomorphometric indices based on digital panoramic and cone beam computed tomography (CBCT) images as osteoporosis predictors in healthy and osteoporotic women. These women had dual Energy x-ray absorptiometry (DEXA) exams and they were categorized

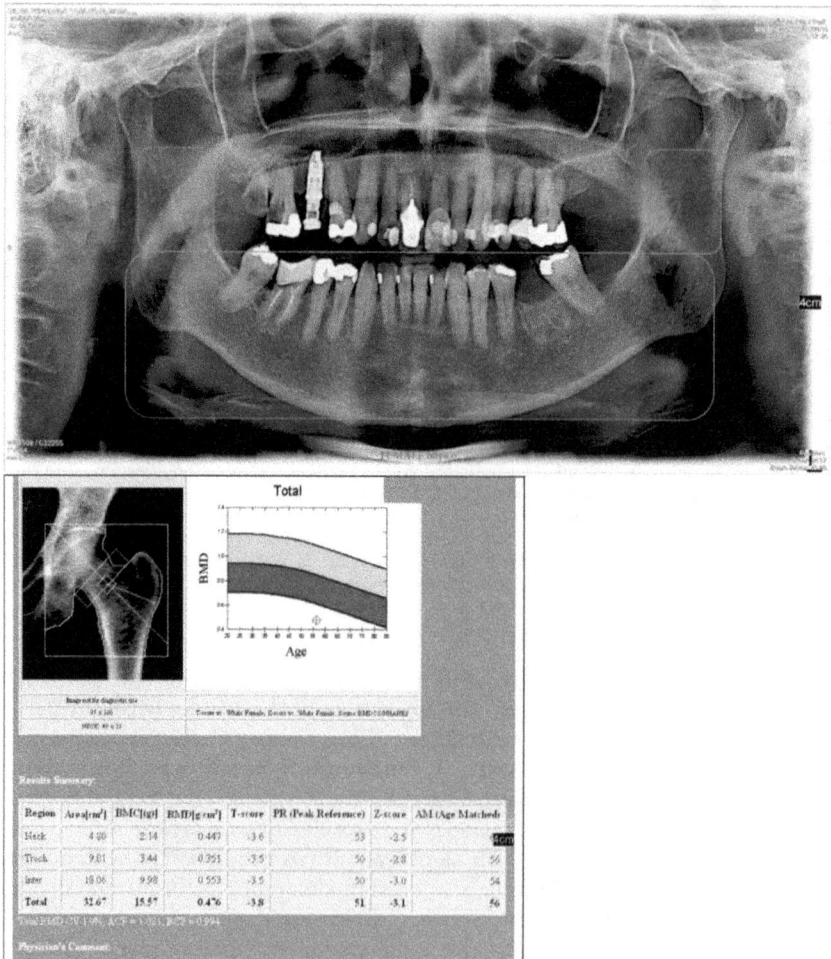

Figure 20.
Panoramic radiography with details on bone quality, of a patient with a T-score pointing to OSTEOPOROSIS on the hip, or femoral head. Note the mandibular bone rarefaction. The mandibular inferior cortex is class II, according to Klemetti. We can also notice the sharp contrast of the oblique line in the retromolar trine on both sides, in addition to the detail of the frame aspect of the cervical vertebrae on the right side.

into either normal or osteopenic/osteoporotic groups. The authors concluded, within the limitation of the yourst study regarding the limited sample size (only 20 patients egyptian females), the bone of the mandible does not appear to reflect the characteristics of the skeleton as a whole [48–49].

About trabecular bone, Barngkgei et al., 2016 studied assessment of jawbone trabecular structure and the dens (the odontoid process of the second cervical vertebra) to test the validity of CBCT among osteoporotic and nonosteoporotic women using CBCT. The authors concluded that the trabecular bone structure of the mandible and maxilla is not affected in osteoporosis as assessed by CBCT. Dens trabecular bone analysis revealed the opposite, so some trabecular bone measures may be assessed by CBCT, which may aid in predicting osteoporosis. These analyzes in CBCT are really difficult to perform, as there are many cuts in each region, which certainly makes it difficult to operate these measures. In the lower cortex of the mandible, this analysis is facilitated due to the small measures involved in the region.

Finally, until the end of 2020, many articles still explored the different indexes and ways of measuring anatomical structures in PAN because it is a wide-ranging examination among the population that is widely used by dentists around the world (**Figures 17–20**).

10. Conclusion

Therefore, this chapter sought to show, through more recent knowledge, the interaction between the oral cavity and osteoporosis and thus demonstrate how the imaging exams used in dentistry can be useful to assess the bone structures of the maxilla and mandible in order to recognize in these structures the signs of low bone mineral density and thus be able to contribute to the diagnosis of osteoporosis, a silent systemic disease that affects most elderly people around the world. We believe that this is a worldwide epidemic with high socio-economic costs, high rates of mortality and morbidity, and therefore, health professionals must work together in this task force to fight osteoporosis.

Conflict of interest

The authors declare no conflict of interest.

Author details

Plauto Christopher Aranha Watanabe[1*], Giovani Antonio Rodrigues[2],
Marcelo Rodrigues Azenha[1], Michel Campos Ribeiro[3],
Enéas de Almeida Souza Filho[3], Rafael Angelo Soares Vieira[3]
and Fabio Santos Bottacin[1]

1 Department of Stomatology, Public Oral Healthy and Forensic Dentistry, Ribeirao
Preto School of Dentistry, University of São Paulo, Brazil

2 Department of Stomatology, School of Dentistry, University of São Paulo, Brazil

3 North College of Minas/FUNORTE, Montes Claros, MG, Brazil

*Address all correspondence to: watanabe@forp.usp.br

IntechOpen

References

[1] S. C. Radominski *et al.*, "Brazilian guidelines for the diagnosis and treatment of postmenopausal osteoporosis," *Rev. Bras. Reumatol. (English Ed.*, vol. 57, no. S 2, pp. 452-466, 2017, doi: 10.1016/j.rbre.2017.07.001.

[2] C. Cooper and *S. Ferrari*, "IOF Compendium of Osteoporosis," *Int. Osteoporos. Found.*, vol. 2nd Editio, pp. 1-76, 2019.

[3] S. A. L. Corrêa, "Editorial," *Semin. Cell Dev. Biol.*, vol. 77, pp. 1-2, 2018, doi: 10.1016/j.semcdb.2017.10.027.

[4] L. O. Monteiro, "Doença Osteometabólica : Aspectos de importância para a população Introdução," pp. 232-243, 2016.

[5] J. E. Compston, M. R. McClung, and W. D. Leslie, "Osteoporosis," *Lancet*, vol. 393, no. 10169, pp. 364-376, 2019, doi: 10.1016/S0140-6736(18)32112-3.

[6] B. Bansal, "Diagnosis of Osteoporosis and Assessment of Fracture Risk," *ESI Man. Clin. Endocrinol.*, vol. 359, pp. 647-647, 2015, doi: 10.5005/jp/books/12535_91.

[7] World Health Organization, "Who Scientific Group on the Assessment of Osteoporosis At Primary Health," *World Health*, vol. May, no. May 2004, pp. 1-13, 2007, doi: 10.1016/S0140-6736(02)08761-5.

[8] J. A. Kanis, "Assessment of fracture risk and its application to screening for postmenopausal osteoporosis: synopsis of a WHO report. WHO Study Group.," *Osteoporos. Int. a J. Establ. as result Coop. between Eur. Found. Osteoporos. Natl. Osteoporos. Found. USA*, vol. 4, no. 6, pp. 368-381, Nov. 1994, doi: 10.1007/BF01622200.

[9] E.-M. Lochmüller, R. Müller, V. Kuhn, C. A. Lill, and F. Eckstein, "Can novel clinical densitometric techniques replace or improve DXA in predicting bone strength in osteoporosis at the hip and other skeletal sites?," *J. bone Miner. Res. Off. J. Am. Soc. Bone Miner. Res.*, vol. 18, no. 5, pp. 906-912, May 2003, doi: 10.1359/jbmr.2003.18.5.906.

[10] L. C. Paiva, S. Filardi, A. M. Pinto-Neto, A. Samara, and J. F. Marques Neto, "Impact of degenerative radiographic abnormalities and vertebral fractures on spinal bone density of women with osteoporosis," *Sao Paulo Med. J.*, vol. 120, no. 1, pp. 9-12, 2002, doi: 10.1590/s1516-31802002000100003.

[11] S. C. Radominski *et al.*, "Diretrizes brasileiras para o diagnóstico e tratamento da osteoporose em mulheres na pós-menopausa," *Rev. Bras. Reumatol.*, vol. 57, no. S 2, pp. 452-466, 2017, doi: 10.1016/j.rbr.2017.06.001.

[12] W. P. Olszynski *et al.*, "Osteoporosis and Treatment in Men : Epidemiology , Prevention ," *Nutrition*, pp. 15-28, 2004.

[13] B. C. G. Marinho, L. P. Guerra, J. B. Drummond, B. C. Silva, and M. M. S. Soares, "The burden of osteoporosis in Brazil.," *Arq. Bras. Endocrinol. Metabol.*, vol. 58, no. 5, pp. 434-443, Jul. 2014, doi: 10.1590/0004-2730000003203.

[14] R. Aziziyeh *et al.*, "The burden of osteoporosis in four Latin American countries: Brazil, Mexico, Colombia, and Argentina.," *J. Med. Econ.*, vol. 22, no. 7, pp. 638-644, Jul. 2019, doi: 10.1080/13696998.2019.1590843.

[15] M. T. E. Guerra, R. D. Viana, L. Feil, E. T. Feron, J. Maboni, and A. S.-G. Vargas, "One-year mortality of elderly patients with hip fracture surgically treated at a hospital in Southern Brazil," *Rev. Bras. Ortop. (English Ed.*, vol. 52, no. 1, pp. 17-23, 2017, doi: 10.1016/j.rboe.2016.11.006.

[16] P. C. A. Watanabe *et al.*, "Morphodigital study of the mandibular trabecular bone in panoramic radiographs," *Int. J. Morphol.*, vol. 25, no. 4, pp. 875-880, 2007, doi: 10.4067/S0717-95022007000400031.

[17] T. H. Lin *et al.*, "Association between periodontal disease and osteoporosis by gender," *Med. (United States)*, vol. 94, no. 7, p. e553, 2015, doi: 10.1097/MD.0000000000000553.

[18] S. Savita, "INTERNATIONAL JOURNAL OF SCIENTIFIC RESEARCH RADIOGRAPHIC COMPARISON OF MANDIBULAR BONE QUALITY IN PATIENTS Periodontology Dr . Benita Maria," no. 1, pp. 27-29, 2019.

[19] G. Jonasson and M. Rythén, "Alveolar bone loss in osteoporosis: A loaded and cellular affair?," *Clin. Cosmet. Investig. Dent.*, vol. 8, pp. 95-103, 2016, doi: 10.2147/CCIDE.S92774.

[20] P. F. van der Stelt, "[Panoramic radiographs in dental diagnostics].," *Ned. Tijdschr. Tandheelkd.*, vol. 123, no. 4, pp. 181-187, Apr. 2016, doi: 10.5177/ntvt.2016.04.15208.

[21] E. Klemetti, S. Kolmakov, and H. Kröger, "Pantomography in assessment of the osteoporosis risk group," *Eur. J. Oral Sci.*, vol. 102, no. 1, pp. 68-72, 1994, doi: 10.1111/j.1600-0722.1994.tb01156.x.

[22] B. Molander, "Panoramic radiography in dental diagnostics.," *Swed. Dent. J. Suppl.*, vol. 119, pp. 1-26, 1996.

[23] B. Cakur, S. Dagistan, A. Sahin, A. Harorli, and A. Yilmaz, "Reliability of mandibular cortical index and mandibular bone mineral density in the detection of osteoporotic women.," *Dentomaxillofac. Radiol.*, vol. 38, no. 5, pp. 255-261, Jul. 2009, doi: 10.1259/dmfr/22559806.

[24] K. Horner and H. Devlin, "The relationships between two indices of mandibular bone quality and bone mineral density measured by dual energy X-ray absorptiometry.," *Dentomaxillofac. Radiol.*, vol. 27, no. 1, pp. 17-21, Jan. 1998, doi: 10.1038/sj.dmfr.4600307.

[25] A. Taguchi, K. Tanimoto, Y. Suei, and T. Wada, "Tooth loss and mandibular osteopenia.," *Oral Surg. Oral Med. Oral Pathol. Oral Radiol. Endod.*, vol. 79, no. 1, pp. 127-132, Jan. 1995, doi: 10.1016/s1079-2104(05)80088-5.

[26] A. Taguchi, K. Tanimoto, Y. Suei, K. Otani, and T. Wada, "Oral signs as indicators of possible osteoporosis in elderly women.," *Oral Surg. Oral Med. Oral Pathol. Oral Radiol. Endod.*, vol. 80, no. 5, pp. 612-616, Nov. 1995, doi: 10.1016/s1079-2104(05)80158-1.

[27] B. W. Benson, T. J. Prihoda, and B. J. Glass, "Variations in adult cortical bone mass as measured by a panoramic mandibular index.," *Oral Surg. Oral Med. Oral Pathol.*, vol. 71, no. 3, pp. 349-356, Mar. 1991, doi: 10.1016/0030-4220(91)90314-3.

[28] E. Calciolari, N. Donos, J. C. Park, A. Petrie, and N. Mardas, "Panoramic measures for oral bone mass in detecting osteoporosis: a systematic review and meta-analysis.," *J. Dent. Res.*, vol. 94, no. 3 Suppl, pp. 17S–27S, Mar. 2015, doi: 10.1177/0022034514554949.

[29] O. S. Kim *et al.*, "Digital panoramic radiographs are useful for diagnosis of osteoporosis in Korean postmenopausal women," *Gerodontology*, vol. 33, no. 2, pp. 185-192, 2016, doi: 10.1111/ger.12134.

[30] T. Alam, I. Alshahrani, K. I. Assiri, S. Almoammar, R. A. Togoo, and M. Luqman, "Evaluation of clinical and radiographic parameters as dental indicators for postmenopausal osteoporosis," *Oral Heal. Prev. Dent.*,

vol. 18, no. 3, pp. 499-504, 2020, doi: 10.3290/j.ohpd.a44688.

[31] C. N. Kato *et al.*, "Use of fractal analysis in dental images: a systematic review.," *Dentomaxillofac. Radiol.*, vol. 49, no. 2, p. 20180457, Feb. 2020, doi: 10.1259/dmfr.20180457.

[32] D. G. Bulut, S. Bayrak, U. Uyeturk, and H. Ankarali, "Mandibular indexes and fractal properties on the panoramic radiographs of the patients using aromatase inhibitors," *Br. J. Radiol.*, vol. 91, no. 1091, 2018, doi: 10.1259/bjr.20180442.

[33] M. D. C. C. Cheade, L. Munhoz, E. S. Arita, and P. C. A. Watanabe, "Opportunistic screening for osteoporosis correlating the bone densities of jaws with multislice computed tomography for cervical vertebrae," *Clin. Lab. Res. Dent.*, no. June, pp. 1-6, 2019, doi: 10.11606/issn.2357-8041.clrd.2019.155263.

[34] M. De Cassia, C. Cheade, A. G. Lourenço, P. Christopher, and A. Watanabe, "Correlation between the Bone Densities Jaws and Cervical Spine through the HU Scale Measured in Multislice Computed Tomography : Opportunistic Screening for Osteoporosis," vol. 2, no. 2, pp. 12-21, 2019.

[35] D. Ledgerton, K. Horner, H. Devlin, and H. Worthington, "Panoramic mandibular index as a radiomorphometric tool: An assessment of precision," *Dentomaxillofacial Radiol.*, vol. 26, no. 2, pp. 95-100, 1997, doi: 10.1038/sj.dmfr.4600215.

[36] E. Klemetti, P. Vainio, V. Lassila, and E. Alhava, "Cortical bone mineral density in the mandible and osteoporosis status in postmenopausal women," *Eur. J. Oral Sci.*, vol. 101, no. 4, pp. 219-223, 1993, doi: 10.1111/j.1600-0722.1993.tb01108.x.

[37] T. E. Southard, K. A. Southard, J. R. Jakobsen, S. L. Hillis, and C. A. Najim, "Fractal dimension in radiographic analysis of alveolar process bone.," *Oral Surg. Oral Med. Oral Pathol. Oral Radiol. Endod.*, vol. 82, no. 5, pp. 569-576, Nov. 1996, doi: 10.1016/s1079-2104(96)80205-8.

[38] T. Nakamoto *et al.*, "Dental panoramic radiograph as a tool to detect postmenopausal women with low bone mineral density: Untrained general dental practitioners' diagnostic performance," *Osteoporos. Int.*, vol. 14, no. 8, pp. 659-664, 2003, doi: 10.1007/s00198-003-1419-y.

[39] S. C. White *et al.*, "Clinical and panoramic predictors of femur bone mineral density.," *Osteoporos. Int. a J. Establ. as result Coop. between Eur. Found. Osteoporos. Natl. Osteoporos. Found. USA*, vol. 16, no. 3, pp. 339-346, Mar. 2005, doi: 10.1007/s00198-004-1692-4.

[40] F. Yaşar and F. Akgünlü, "The differences in panoramic mandibular indices and fractal dimension between patients with and without spinal osteoporosis," *Dentomaxillofacial Radiol.*, vol. 35, no. 1, pp. 1-9, 2006, doi: 10.1259/dmfr/97652136.

[41] P. C. A. Watanabe, F. C. Dias, J. P. M. Issa, S. A. C. Monteiro, F. J. A. De Paula, and R. Tiossi, "Elongated styloid process and atheroma in panoramic radiography and its relationship with systemic osteoporosis and osteopenia," *Osteoporos. Int.*, vol. 21, no. 5, pp. 831-836, 2010, doi: 10.1007/s00198-009-1022-y.

[42] A. Taguchi, "Triage screening for osteoporosis in dental clinics using panoramic radiographs," *Oral Dis.*, vol. 16, no. 4, pp. 316-327, 2010, doi: 10.1111/j.1601-0825.2009.01615.x.

[43] A. F. Leite, P. T. de S. Figueiredo, C. M. Guia, N. S. Melo, and A. P. de Paula,

"Correlations between seven panoramic radiomorphometric indices and bone mineral density in postmenopausal women," *Oral Surgery, Oral Med. Oral Pathol. Oral Radiol. Endodontology*, vol. 109, no. 3, pp. 449-456, 2010, doi: 10.1016/j.tripleo.2009.02.028.

[44] H. Devlin and C. Whelton, "Can mandibular bone resorption predict hip fracture in elderly women? A systematic review of diagnostic test accuracy," *Gerodontology*, vol. 32, no. 3, pp. 163-168, 2015, doi: 10.1111/ger.12077.

[45] L. Munhoz, A. R. G. Cortes, and E. S. Arita, "Assessment of osteoporotic alterations in type 2 diabetes: A retrospective study," *Dentomaxillofacial Radiol.*, vol. 46, no. 6, pp. 1-5, 2017, doi: 10.1259/dmfr.20160414.

[46] C. C. Gomes, G. L. De Rezende Barbosa, R. P. Bello, F. N. Bóscolo, and S. M. De Almeida, "A comparison of the mandibular index on panoramic and cross-sectional images from CBCT exams from osteoporosis risk group," *Osteoporos. Int.*, vol. 25, no. 7, pp. 1885-1890, 2014, doi: 10.1007/s00198-014-2696-3.

[47] M. B. C. C. Alonso, T. V. Vasconcelos, L. J. Lopes, P. C. A. Watanabe, and D. Q. Freitas, "Validation of cone-beam computed tomography as a predictor of osteoporosis using the Klemetti classification.," *Braz. Oral Res.*, vol. 30, no. 1, May 2016, doi: 10.1590/1807-3107BOR-2016.vol30.0073.

[48] A. J. Camargo, A. R. G. Cortes, E. M. Aoki, M. G. Baladi, E. S. Arita, and P. C. A. Watanabe, "Diagnostic performance of fractal dimension and radiomorphometric indices from digital panoramic radiographs for screening low bone mineral density," *Brazilian J. Oral Sci.*, vol. 15, no. 2, pp. 131-136, 2016, doi: 10.20396/bjos.v15i2.8648764.

[49] C. W. Jeong, K. H. Kim, H. W. Jang, H. S. Kim, and J. K. Huh, "The relationship between oral tori and bite force," *Cranio - J. Craniomandib. Pract.*, vol. 37, no. 4, pp. 246-253, 2019, doi: 10.1080/08869634.2017.1418617.